ALCOHOLISM AND THE BRAIN

Dedicated to Marty Mann,
who has done more in educating, understanding and treating alcoholism than all the medical profession

ALCOHOLISM AND THE BRAIN

A. E. BENNETT, M.D.
The A. E. Bennett Neuropsychiatric Foundation
Berkeley, California

Stratton Intercontinental Medical Book Corp. / New York

LC 76-54392. ISBN 0-913258-45-8

Printed in U.S.A.

CONTENTS

FOREWORD

As the fine neurologist and psychiatrist that he is, Dr. A. E. Bennett has often stressed the effects of alcohol upon the brain. While many books have been written about alcoholism, in general, including one edited by this writer ("Alcoholism," Charles C Thomas, Publisher, 1956), it remained for Dr. Bennett to produce a book in which specific facets of brain function are considered in relation to alcoholism as a brain disease.

The book is divided into eight chapters, and six of these are concerned specifically with the effects of alcohol upon the nervous system, particularly the brain. In fact the word "brain" appears in four chapter titles and "neuropathology" in one other. The author postulates that alcoholism is a brain disease of itself and that it causes other brain diseases. The human being drinks alcohol because he has a brain, and his excesses with alcohol impair his brain.

In his chapter on "Psychiatric Alcoholic Brain Disorders," Dr. Bennett has provided a masterful survey of alcoholic illnesses which affect every aspect of human existence. Statistics are almost meaningless where alcoholism is concerned, but it is probably safe to say that some aspect of alcoholism affects nearly every family.

Dr. Bennett speaks of alcoholism and epilepsy and the importance of the alcoholic epileptic disorders. He concurs with this writer's concept that Acute Pathological Alcoholic Intoxication is an acute alcoholic brain syndrome and is identical with psychomotor epilepsy, except that it is triggered by alcohol. The tremendous importance of this syndrome in medicolegal cases has been emphasized.

Perhaps in no other writing except Dr. Bennett's papers has the syndrome of the intermediate stage of alcoholic brain disease been so clearly elucidated and stressed. The author points out the frequency with which this syndrome is encountered by physicians yet not recognized, the frequency with which the patient struggles against this illness, not receiving medical help. The writer concurs fully with Dr. Bennett that alcoholism is a disease, and, as he points out, usually progressive. It is long-term in duration and there is deterioration through its progress and consequences. Quantitative studies have been able to present only estimates of the size and scope of the problem.

The report of the World Health Organization's Expert Committee in this field states: "At present the fact must be faced that very few countries know even the extent of the problem created by the grossest form of this disorder [alcoholism].'' It examined with interest the Jellinek Estimation Formula, which, since its use in the United States, has been applied to other countries.

Of interest is the title of a newly published book, ''Chemical Coping,''* which includes alcohol among other legal drugs which are used by people who habitually use chemicals to manage their lives or ''cope'' with those situations which life itself brings to all of us. It is stated that no one knows the personal and social benefits derived from such chemical management and coping as compared with the costs associated with such adapting behavior. Here is another implication of the widespread use of alcohol and the reasons and needs behind that use.

The author of ''Alcoholism and the Brain'' is a man of so many accomplishments that they cannot be listed here. He was born in Alliance, Nebraska, January 12, 1898, and obtained the Bachelor of Science and Medical Doctorate degrees from the University of Nebraska. His postgraduate training was taken at Philadelphia General Hospital and John Hopkins University. Dr. Bennett practiced in Omaha, Nebraska from 1924 to 1948.

He organized the A. E. Bennett Neuropsychiatric Research Foundation in 1942 and has been its continuing director since that time. This is a nonprofit Foundation that has contributed immeasurably through the years to the advancement of research in Neurology and Psychiatry.

Dr. Bennett is a Fellow of the American Psychiatric Association, The American Medical Association, The Association for the Advancement of Science, and is Past-President and Honorary Member of the Society of Biological Psychiatry. In 1970, the latter Society awarded him its Gold Medal for noteworthy contributions to the field of Biological Psychiatry.

He was Chairman and Professor of Neurology and Psychiatry at the University of Nebraska College of Medicine and Associate Clinical Professor of Psychiatry, University of California at Berkeley. He is Consultant in Neurology and Psychiatry to the Veterans Administration. He has received meritorious awards from the American Medical Association for research in ''Crude Curare,'' ''Myasthenia and Curarization'' and ''Alcohol Brain Disease.''

Dr. Bennett pioneered the development of psychiatric treatment in general hospitals and developed the A. E. Bennett Psychiatric Pavilion at the Herrick Memorial Hospital, Berkeley, California in 1947.

He is the author of 250 articles on neurology and psychiatry and of a textbook entitled, ''Psychiatric Nursing Technique''. He is author of a book entitled, "The Practice of Psychiatry in General Hospitals.''

Dr. Bennett is a man of many interests that range from hunting and fishing

* Chambers, C. D. et al.: Chemical Coping: A report on legal drugs in the U.S. New York, Halstead Press, 1975.

to farming. He is the father of three fine children. The central theme of his life has been the progress of research in Neurology and Psychiatry, and in 1974 he published what is essentially an autobiography, a book entitled "Fifty Years in Neurology and Psychiatry."

His interests during the past several years have expanded the knowledge and interests of doctors from other lands in the advancement of his chosen fields, and specifically of Biological Psychiatry. The present book is an example and product of this consuming interest. Research workers in these areas will be indebted to Dr. Bennett for his production of this treatise, which should be of great interest to psychiatrists, neurologists, neurochemists, neuropathologists, psychologists, social workers, members of the judiciary and of law enforcement agencies, all those interested in the field of foresic psychiatry and in fact all other students of the medical and legal arts and of the humanities.

George N. Thompson, M.D.

INTRODUCTION

It is estimated that between five and ten million, or about five per cent, of the people in the United States are victims of alcoholism. It is on the increase, 200,000 yearly. For example, over twenty per cent of admissions to California State Hospitals are diagnosed as alcoholism. Once an alcoholic becomes a compulsive drinker he cannot stop unaided. He becomes addicted. This is our nation's number one addictive disorder and a major public health problem. If all the complications from alcoholic abuse were correctly evaluated in our vital statistics—such as liver cirrhosis, alcoholic brain disease, pancreatitis, gastritis, cardiac myopathies, suicides, accidental deaths—it would be the third cause of death.* The morbidity in shortening life (10–12 years), handicapping in one's employment, skid row types with malnutrition and its effect on secondary diseases, often fatal and other factors have never been adequately correlated.

Despite the fact that all the evidence indicates a progressively fatal outcome for the compulsive heavy drinker, articles continue to question whether alcoholism is a symptom or a disease. Most articles place the emphasis on psychological and social aspects of the problem, with little emphasis upon the most important part, namely the effect of too much alcohol upon the nervous system. The first report, "Alcohol and Alcoholism," by the United States Department of Health, Education and Welfare (1967) gave no adequate discussion of the importance of alcoholic brain disease. In most symposia on alcohol there are few if any papers on alcohol as an addictive disorder, which is the most important aspect of the problem, because the alcoholic becomes dependent from brain damage. Extensive research over the past twenty-five years in this area seems to have been overlooked by most writers on alcohol. The major emphasis is that alcoholism is indicative of an underlying personality disorder. The facts are that after sustained heavy drinking over a period of years, organic brain damage occurs, causing loss of control over one's drinking; this calls for medical management first, treating the addictive disorder. After obtaining complete abstinence, then, if a psychiatric disorder or social maladjustment is found to exist, this must be treated appropriately.

This monograph has been prepared to give at least some counterbalance to the heavy emphasis on the view of chronic alcoholism as of social psychogenic cause rather than considering the effects of an addictive toxic drug upon cerebral function and its resultant behavior disorders. In spite of the many failures

* An editorial in the AMA Newsletter of March 3, 1975 (p. 4) states: "At least 100,000 deaths a year are alcohol related."

of psychotherapy in treating alcoholism, it is still being advocated by many psychiatrists, either by individual therapy or in groups. The disease, alcoholism, then continues its progressive course because the addictive disorder has not been brought under control.

In the following pages I attempt a comprehensive accumulation of data about neurologic disorders deriving from the toxic effects of alcohol, along with secondary pathologic effects. The topics that are covered are the pharmacologic, neurophysiologic and neuropathologic effects of alcohol on the nervous system; the clinical psychiatric neurologic disorders and stages of alcoholic brain disease; evaluating diagnostic aids, clinical, psychological, electroencephalographic, pneumoencephalographic, computer brain scan in brain damages; the problems in rehabilitation and the reasons for failure in the management of compulsive addictive alcoholics.

The character disorder from chronic alcoholism shows itself in intellectual impairment, judgment defects, loss of mental efficiency, with general progressive deterioration in global functioning ability. These personality changes are due to brain damage and thus do not respond to psychotherapy.

The large majority of writers on alcoholism are biochemists, physiologists, anatomists, sociologists and psychologists. There is a paucity of articles by practitioners of medicine who really study and treat severely ill alcoholics. Much of what is written is of little practical value in prevention of the disease, and the treatment or rehabilitation of the millions of alcoholics. Because of this, fifteen to twenty per cent of our private patients have been alcoholics. We have devoted a major effort for years to interest the medical profession further in facing up to the problem.

This effort has in turn led us into investigations into the role of alcoholic addiction and the brain diseases, both neurologic and psychiatric aspects. We established the first psychiatric unit in a general community hospital in California which opened up its beds to alcoholics, one of the few general hospitals at that time that admitted alcoholics. Our researchers, after several scientific exhibits before the American Medical Association, The American Psychiatric Association and other societies, finally led to the first award from the A.M.A. (1956) for research in alcoholism for investigations in alcoholic brain disease.

Another aim has been to get more physicians to better understand and help salvage disabled victims of alcoholism and also to overcome the false impression of poor prognosis in the treatment of the chronic alcoholic. This led to my establishing of annual scholarships to attend a summer school on alcoholism at Rutgers University, hoping to interest more young practitioners, who are so greatly needed in alcoholic rehabilitative programs.

Another purpose, at the same time, has been to bring about a better and more understanding relationship between Alcoholics Anonymous groups and physicians who are treating alcoholics.

In a conference on alcoholism and the central nervous system held in 1973, the most comprehensive symposium ever held on this aspect of the disease at that time, Dr. Frank A. Seixas, conference chairman, in his introductory remarks stated: "It is a curious fact that this type of conference has not been held before, despite the obvious fact that the reason anybody drinks is to get the effect of the action of alcohol on the central nervous system, and much of the major pathology of heavy drinking is well known to be neurological." He further elaborated that the conference was to examine critically and analyze ethanol action on the brain, its chemical basis, and the chemical basis for tolerance, withdrawal and reproduction of the phenomena in animals. Also to be examined were electroencephalographic changes, new research, and how ethanol destroys brain tissue, producing the chronic organic syndromes—but there was nothing about treatment or the importance of alcoholic psychiatric disorders in the symposium. My great concern (and another reason for this monograph) is to get a fuller understanding of the complex problems of alcoholism, with thus better medical and psychiatric management of its serious complications. I consider the principal complication to be involvement of the brain. Future research in this area should be of top priority, along with prevention of the disease by early detection of addiction-prone patients.

Hopefully this monograph will be an aid to those seriously concerned with understanding the myriad problems and the treatment of alcoholism.

CHAPTER ONE

Alcoholism as a Disease

E. M. Jellinek, considered a pioneer researcher and authority on alcoholism, covers the subject in his book, "The Disease Concept of Alcoholism,"* up to 1960. This volume completely covers the history and development of the medical concept of alcoholism as a disease, which culminated in the American Medical Association's resolution in 1956 to declare alcoholism a medical illness. Because of his pioneer investigations, physicians recently have been advocating changing the name of alcoholism to "Jellinek's disease."

Jellinek formulated different types of alcoholism under Greek letter symbols, alpha, beta, gamma, delta, epsilon. The *alpha types* are individuals with purely psychological dependence, where alcohol is used to relieve emotional tensions but with the ability to abstain, with no loss of control and no signs of progressive disease, even after thirty to forty years of drinking (although many of them do change into the gamma alcoholic type).

Beta alcoholism: This is considered alcoholism with complications of such systemic diseases as gastritis, cirrhosis, and polyneuritis. These occur from excess alcohol plus nutritional deficiency factors and may occur without physical or psychological dependency on alcohol, but these persons also can progress to gamma or delta alcoholism.

Gamma alcoholism: This characterizes addictive types that acquire tissue tolerance to alcohol, withdrawal symptoms, and craving with physiologic dependence and loss of control. These individuals also show marked behavioral personality changes. This is the phase that I have described as alcoholic brain damage in the intermediate stage of alcoholic brain disease [1]. Gamma alcoholism is apparently the predominant species of alcoholism in the United States and Canada and in other Anglo-Saxon countries.

Delta alcoholism has the characteristics of gamma alcoholism, but besides loss of control and inability to abstain, these persons "have no ability to go on the wagon" without withdrawal symptoms. I contend this phase is true physiologic addiction, and loss of control comes from brain damage.

Epsilon alcoholism is characterized by periodic alcoholism, including serious physical damage with each bout, but the individual is able to resist drinking for a few months at a time.

Jellinek does not classify the more advanced stage of alcoholism, resulting in permanent brain damage as we see in Korsakoff's-Wernicke's disease. He com-

---

* University Press, New Haven, Conn., and Hillhouse Press, New Brunswick, N.J., 1960 and 1962.

pares other drug addictions similar to alcohol with dependency loss of control "caused by physio-pathological processes as diseases."

Jellinek believed that heavy drinking is not entirely due to psychological or social factors. In the later stages there is a physiologic factor which accounts for the disease condition and is outwardly manifested mostly by loss of control. Little and McAvoy, in 1952 [2], electroencephalographic studies, postulated that there are changes in the cerebral condition that predispose to alcoholism. Leveboullet, in 1954 [3], stated that brain damage from alcohol plus nutritional factors can explain to a large extent the essential pathology of alcoholism, namely the permanent loss of control. Jellinek elaborated 31 other theories by various authors. Six are chemical or endocrinologic, some are based on allergy, nutritional factors are emphasized by many, but only two of the authorities mention brain damage as an important factor in alcoholism.

In discussing brain pathology, Jellinek cites the pioneer work of Courville [4] and Meyers [5] in 1954, Bennett, Doi, and Mowrey in 1956 on electroencephalographic changes [6], and especially the work of Fred Lemere [7], who in 1956 postulated specific alcoholic brain changes. Jellinek concluded that there is a lack of evidence that these brain changes relate to the etiology of alcoholism, but he considered the hypothesis that brain damage may be responsible for loss of control over drinking and the production of characteristic behavioral changes. This is the only place in which Jellinek really approaches our ideas of the basic cause of loss of control in alcoholism. He also noted at least six investigators who cited EEG changes and pneumoencephalographic changes of cortical atrophy since 1952.

Lemere, more than the others, however, has taken a more positive stand since 1956 in favor of an etiology of alcoholic addiction founded on cerebral cortical atrophy (probably based on Courville's work), along with the indirect effects of nutritional deficiencies. He believes, as we do, that the permanent loss of control over drinking comes from cellular damage (atrophy) from progressive destruction of the frontal cortex. These centers are the most subjected to the effects of alcohol, and in the confirmed addict, once alcohol enters his system, there is an immediate paralysis of the control centers of the brain and permanent loss of drinking control. Sudden withdrawal produces cellular craving for alcohol. Lemere [8] has also more recently postulated that sexual impotence resulting from excessive alcoholic intake is on an organic basis.

Other researchers, notably Mardones [9] and Williams [10] have written extensively on the nutritional etiology of alcoholism. They have elaborated this along with a genetotrophic theory, much of it based upon animal experimentation in nutritional anomalies and biochemical and metabolic deficiencies, in an attempt to explain the craving or physical need for alcohol. Williams [10] elaborated a theory that an alcoholic suffers from an abnormal craving because of an inherited metabolic fault which causes his body to require certain elements in great excess over the normal. These are also important factors in the complications of alcoholic systemic diseases—cirrhosis, pancreatitis, gastritis and related neurologic lesions—but these secondary complications do not of themselves adequately explain the process of alcoholic addiction.

Likewise, others have advanced an endocrinologic etiology for alcoholism. "Repeated exposure to stress results in repeated adrenal stimulation and eventually glandular exhaustion."* Gonadal factors also derive from malnutrition. Again these are consequences of systemic diseases from alcohol without explaining the addictive process—namely, the craving and loss of control and compulsive drinking pattern with acquired tolerance, and withdrawal symptoms; all of these are physiologic addictive symptoms.

Jellinek further cites 22 authorities on alcoholism who have formulated theories of alcoholism as a pharmacologic process of addiction. Many compare it with narcotic addiction and barbital. Also dependency from prolonged excessive drinking seems to occur without neurotic basis, but only two authors in this group speak of metabolic cellular disturbances in the brain as part of the etiology of addiction. None stresses the fact that the alcoholic addict frequently easily slips into other drug addictions, with thus multiple addictions. Any analgesic or sedative drug is an additional hazard for the alcoholic.

Physicians generally are not sufficiently aware of how alcoholic addiction develops. They are not taught in medical schools. Many dislike to treat alcoholics, and the medical profession itself has one of the highest incidences of alcoholism.† Psychiatrists generally still rely too much on the psychological interpretation of the symptoms of alcoholic abuse, and even delirium tremens is ignored as a distinct symptom of physiologic withdrawal, similar to narcotic or barbital intoxication.

Jellinek summarizes the pros and cons for psychological versus physiologic addiction. "In spite of the great diversity of personality structures among alcoholics, there appears in a large proportion a low tolerance for tension with inability to cope with physiological stresses. For such people, they may be induced to use larger quantities with such frequency that pharmacological, physical dependent addiction is facilitated." This still does not explain fully the etiology, since it neglects the importance of the effect of alcohol upon cerebral function and resultant behavioral personality changes.

N. Bejerot has published a book, "Addiction and Artificially Induced Disease" (Charles C Thomas, Publishers 1972), in which he states his view that addiction results from the use of a drug over a sufficient period rather than

---

* Goldfarb, A. J., Berman, S.: Alcoholism as a psychosomatic disorder. Quart. J. Alcoholism 10: 415–429, 1949.

† "Physicians suffer the highest rate of alcoholism of any profession and are not aware of the gradual insidious addictive qualities." Council on Mental Health: JAMA 223: 684, 1975.

from social or psychological maladjustments. In treatment, concentration on amelioration of any initial emotional difficulty without starting with the drug abuse problem and controlling it first will not effectively treat the addictive process. The addict acquires a desire to drink as strong as an instinctual drive. He may seek help of a dependency nature, but seldom is willing to give up the drug. Bejerot recommends compulsory treatment, extensive control with close aftercare and the use of psychotherapy, and facilitating new occupational and social adjustments and education to get the patient motivated to control the addictive process. This often requires a new environment, with removal away from all temptation and other alcoholics who might induce relapse.

So far as the brain is concerned, it is logical to assume that there is a progressive destruction of the frontal cortex with resultant disorders in function of will power, judgment and control. Eventually the stage is reached where small amounts of alcohol result in loss of control. Few alcoholics intend to drink too much, but once alcohol enters the body there occurs immediate paralysis of the control centers in the brain, and the helpless alcoholic can't stop until he is unconscious. This is why true alcoholic addicts must never take one drink, as they always revert to the uncontrolled pattern of drinking. The evidence for these postulates is given in the following chapters.

The current orientation of most psychiatrists to alcoholism is to consider alcoholism as a symptom of some underlying condition so they do not treat it as a disease itself. Consequently, psychotherapy is directed toward the underlying disturbance. Unsatisfactory results of psychiatry have been explained on the basis of the severity of the underlying personality disorder. This is fallacious rationalization. Alcoholic addiction usually does involve an underlying personality disorder, but once addicted, the patient has the added factor of a chronic toxic state due to constant alcohol exposure. The character disorder that occurs is organically determined and will not respond to psychotherapy. Judgment defects and loss in mental efficiency are evidence of intellectual impairment. These and other personality changes make the victim unable to integrate at higher functioning levels. The organic nature cannot easily be determined in the early stages of brain damage. All patients after an acute alcoholic episode should have a complete evaluating diagnosis to determine the degree of organic residual systemic and cerebral changes. The ways to do this are covered in Chapters Four and Six.

CHAPTER TWO

Pharmacology and Physiologic Action of Alcohol on the Brain

The Mode of Action of Alcohol

The immediate primary effect of alcohol is narcotic, inhibiting function of nerve cells that are especially sensitive to its action, and prolonged action occurs because of the high lipoid content of accumulating alcohol. This is shown by the high alcohol content in the brain in fatal cases. This narcotic action resembles that of anoxia.

Alcohol is metabolized in the brain, as well as in the liver, to acetylaldehyde and acetic acid, which are products of oxidation by the brain. Alcohol is quickly transferred by the blood stream directly to brain tissues; passing through the cell membranes, it modifies the consistency of the protoplasm in the cells. At first the action tends to increase cell permeability, inhibiting conduction of electrical changes on the membrane surface. In greater concentration there is decreasing permeability, if long continued, resulting in cell death. The complex reaction is due to a number of factors: nutritional deficiency, anoxic effects, associated metabolic poisons and associated conditions such as blood sludging. Alcohol interferes with the metabolism of the nerve cells, largely from modifying viscosity, liquifying protoplasm and in larger concentrations resulting in coagulation and cell death. All this is associated with nutritional factors, oxygenation, vitamin B_1 deficiency and glucose metabolism, but direct specific action of narcotic alcohol starts the process of disturbance in cellular metabolism. Secondary effects are circulatory changes, with congestion and hemorrhages resulting from stagnation from slowing down of the blood vessel current (blood sludging). This results in anoxia. The anoxic action reinforces the narcotic action, paving the way for cell death and finally cerebral atrophy.

Shortly after ingestion of alcohol it becomes present in the cerebrospinal fluid at lower concentrations than in the blood, but as the blood level falls, the cerebrospinal fluid concentration remains high. Alcohol is metabolized at the rate of ten to twenty mg. an hour, so that if one would drink only about an ounce of whiskey an hour he would never become intoxicated. The compulsive drinker, however, usually consumes several drinks within an hour. The individual effects vary greatly, dependent upon many factors, such as tolerance, weight, amount of food previously ingested, and the general health of the person (for example, following a gastrectomy only a small amount can be tolerated).

Alcohol is a high-energy food, combining chemical properties of glucose and ether, which acts quickly but cannot be stored. Alcohol produces heat energy but is not capable of supplying nutritional needs. It contains no vitamins or essential amino acids, and since these are required for the metabolism of alcohol, there is a constant nutritional disorder present in chronic alcoholics. The steps of oxidation in the liver is oxidation to acetylaldehyde by an enzyme, alcohol dehydrogenase (ADH), which utilizes nicotinamide adenine dinucleotide (NAD); ultimately the end products are carbon dioxide and water.

The Effects of Alcohol upon the Brain

Depression of the nervous system is the principal action. The first mental processes affected are those dealing with self-restraint. In general, the central nervous system effects are proportional to the blood alcohol level. In higher levels the anesthetic effect takes over, lasting for several hours. The exact biochemical explanation of neurochemical interactions is not known. It is known that serotonin and other biogenic amines such as dopamine greatly potentiate the central nervous system effects of alcohol and these effects may be mediated through biogenic amines. Certain investigators have postulated that acetylaldehyde alters dopamine metabolism, producing metabolites that could be the basis of the addictive process. Such an hypothesis is not proved but does deserve further research.

Since the principal effect of alcohol is as a central nervous system depressant, there is potentiation upon the use of sedative, hypnotic and tranquilizing drugs that are either multiple addictive or synergistic. This is extremely important in treatment, and also in the prevention of overdose or possible suicide.

Disufiram and calcium carbamide, when combined with alcohol, block aldehyde dehydrogenase, needed for alcohol metabolism. This leads to a large increase in acetylaldehyde which shows itself first by throbbing in the head from vasodilatation, with severe flushing, sweating, pallor, dropping blood pressure, nausea, dyspnea, chest pain, palpitation, even syncopy and collapse. The severity of the symptoms depends upon the alcohol blood level and the amount of drug ingested, but it is an excellent physiologic blocking agent, of great value in the management of chronic, compulsive alcoholic addiction (Chapter Eight).

Other conditions related to alcohol include the effects on carbohydrate metabolism. Hepatic glycogenolysis is augmented after ingestion of alcohol, producing hypoglycemia. Liver disease, pancreatitis and malnutrition predispose to alcoholic hypoglycemia. Thus there is need for intravenous glucose in acute alcoholic intoxication states. There is a deficiency in magnesium, and the fall of blood serum magnesium correlates with neuromuscular hyperexcitability in the withdrawal stage of alcoholism and may be responsible for the convulsive seizures so often followed by delirium tremens. With the reduced rates of flow through the capillaries caused by the sludged blood, the tissues between the capillaries are deprived of oxygen. Also, as the rate of the flow decreases, there is a decrease in the delivery of glucose to the intercapillary neurons. In addition, acid radicals accumulate and the tissue disintegration products are not carried away from the anoxic hypoglycemic areas, thus producing local acidosis. The altered behavior and mental deterioration in habitual drinkers is attributed to the minute volumes of tissue in the nervous system that suffer from stagnant anoxia. These changes have also been demonstrated in animals, resulting from ethanol agglutination of the blood cells and forcible reduction of the flow rates plugging the vessels. When these animals are preheparinized, the blood does not agglutinate, even with lethal doses of alcohol [11,12]. These important studies help explain the mechanism of alcoholic brain disease, along with the observations of Courville and others on the biochemical effects and the direct toxic effect of alcohol upon the nerve cells, resulting finally in atrophy of the brain.

Blomstrand [13] of Sweden studied the effects of pyrazole in slowing down ethanol metabolism in the liver, in explanation of the mechanism of fatty liver leading to cirrhosis. He feels that other metabolic disturbances associated with alcoholism can likewise be explained, such as the effects of alcohol on the central nervous system. Liver changes are seen in fifty per cent of autopsies in cases of alcoholic cerebral atrophy. True liver cirrhosis has been produced experimentally in dogs and rabbits by feeding adequate diets along with excess alcohol [14]. The evidence is convincing that alcohol alone can cause cirrhosis.

Rubin and Lieber [14], recently reported a long term study on alcohol ingestion along with a nutritious diet in producing liver disease in baboons. All developed fatty livers, alcoholic hepatitis or cirrhosis. They conclude that alcohol is the toxin. Two animals developed delirium tremens when they stopped eating. These studies should be correlated with neuropathology of the brain, as Courville has shown that fifty per cent of cerebral atrophy cases had associated liver disease. The term hepatogenic encephalopathy has been ascribed to some cases of alcoholic brain disease where there is marked liver disease, and there must be some relationship. This is a potentially fruitful field for research to better understand alcoholic brain disorders.

The idea that pharmacologic and emotional factors combine to cause memory distortion that inclines the alcoholic to deny his condition cannot be substantiated. The evidence is that organic brain changes cause memory distortion, loss of insight and change in personality, and that these cause the addicted alcoholic to deny his dependency.

CHAPTER THREE

Neuropathology of Alcoholism

This chapter is largely a condensation from the classic book by Cyril B. Courville, "The Effects of Alcoholism on the Nervous System of Man" (San Lucas Press, Los Angeles, 1955).

I should add that this monumental work was largely responsible for our researches in the field of early diagnosis of alcoholic brain disease. In our scientific exhibits before the American Medical Association in 1956 and 1957 on alcoholic brain disease we had one panel of pictures donated by Dr. Courville on neuropathologic observations which depicted the atrophy of the brain and microscopic findings. When Dr. Courville viewed our efforts, he complimented us on our complete clinical application to his basic anatomic studies. We were given a scientific award from the A.M.A., the first ever given for research in alcoholism.

From thousands of autopsy examinations at Los Angeles County Hospital, Courville selected 124 confirmed chronic alcoholics and observed that the great majority of cases showed the cortical atrophy consistently occurring in chronic alcoholism. He extended his studies to get a complete picture of the neuropathology of alcoholism, including Wernicke's syndrome, encephalitis, hemorrhagica superior, described in 1881. The latter was the first described structural disorder with focal hemorrhage in the nuclear gray matter in the walls of the aqueduct, third and fourth ventricles.

In Wernicke's original cases, chronic alcoholism was the etiologic factor. Subsequently, during the period 1880 to 1900, a number of investigators described such changes as degenerative changes or thickened meninges, alterations in optic nerves and cortical cells in alcoholics. These investigators were reporting nerve cell changes in such conditions as alcoholic pellagra, changes in the spinal cord and peripheral neuropathies, and finally the degeneration of the corpus callosum (Marchiafava-Bignami disease) and cerebellar atrophy in chronic alcoholism.

According to Courville's description, gross and cellular damage occurs in acute alcoholic intoxication and in delirium tremens. He describes gross changes as principally brain edema (wet brain) with excessive amounts of cerebrospinal fluid, congestion of the pial and central blood vessels with petechial hemorrhages, and in some cases extravasation of blood.

The microscopic alterations are of nerve cells, the ependyma and choroid plexus, along with swelling changes of blood vessels and edematous changes showing vascular dilatation and engorgement; also occurring are diapedesis from capillaries with perivascular edema and similar changes in the ependyma and choroid plexus. In fatal delirium tremens there are similar findings, but also more chronic changes, such as thickening of the leptomeninges with varying degrees of frontal cortical atrophy and enlargement of the ventricles. There is microscopic progressive deterioration with loss of pyramidal cells along with acute swelling of the large deep layer of pyramidal cells. The changes are principally in cell cytoplasm and deformed dendrites (Fig. 1). These changes are most conspicuous in the frontal, central and parietal cortex. Also, changes are seen in the nerve cells of the basal ganglia regions, with demylenization of fibers and changes in interstitial cells described. Purkinji cells of the cerebellum show loss of cellular substance, with progressive deterioration.

Special organic cerebral disease syndromes are delineated as to their pathology. The hemorrhagic encephalopathy of Wernicke-Korsakoff's syndrome is usually due to continuation of chronic alcoholism plus vitamin defi-

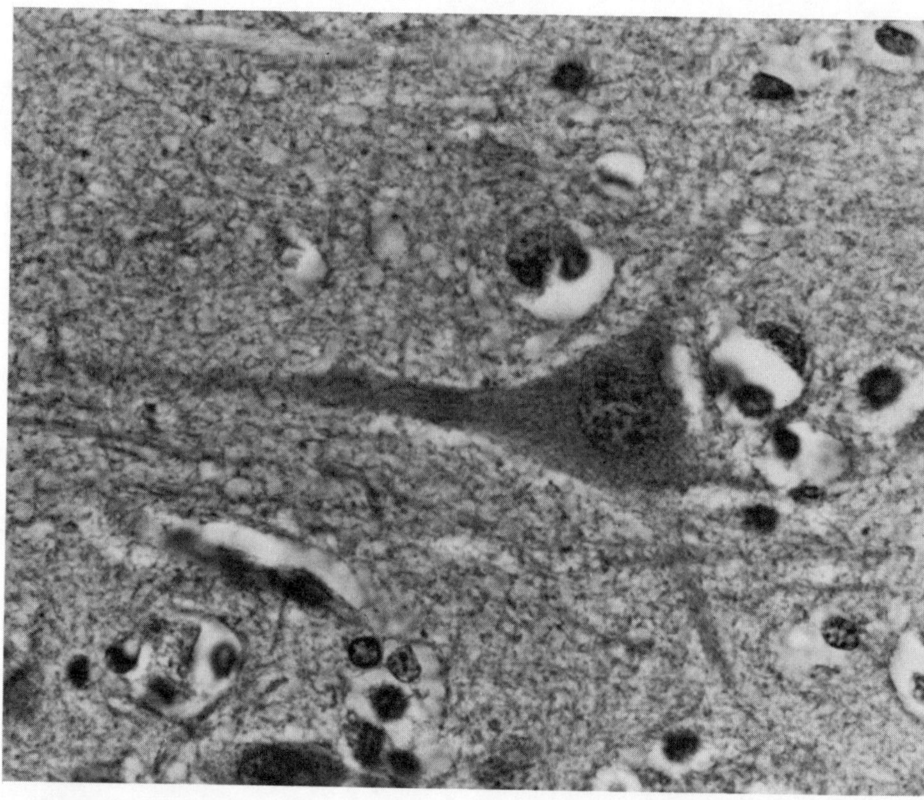

FIG. 1. Deterioration of pyramidal elements—ghost cells—widened pericellular spaces—halos about oligodendrocytes.

ciency. This condition has been produced experimentally in rats and pigeons. The principal pathologic changes occur in the mamillary bodies, hypothalamic nuclei, peri-aqueductal gray matter, the ocolomotor nuclei and areas in the midbrain. The primary histologic alterations consist of vascular changes with secondary degeneration of regional nerve and interstitial cells. There are some areas of small perivascular and larger hemorrhagic areas resulting in degeneration of cell bodies. There are also frequently associated spinal cord and peripheral neuropathies.

Alcoholic Atrophy of the Cerebral Cortex

This is the most pertinent chapter in Courville's book and the one that lays the groundwork for a real understanding of progressive alcoholic encephalopathy. After repeated alcoholic exposures or constant excessive drinking, there results a progressive atrophy of the frontal lobes. This is most prominently seen in the dorsal lateral convolutions. It is seen most commonly in the fifth and sixth decades but also has been described as early as the fourth decade.

The gross pathology shows uniform atrophy of convolutions (Figs. 2 and 3), extending from the upper part to the middle and lower areas, including the pre- and post-central gyri and also the superior parietal lobes. There is associated thickening and opacities of the overlying meninges. The degree of atrophy is not as severe as seen in senility.

There is also a syndrome that has been called alcoholic pseudo-paresis which shows itself as a progressive intellectual impairment with distinctive personality changes. Here the sulci are filled with fluid when drained and air replaced, the process can be visualized by pneumogram, which displays the cortical atrophy and the dilated subarachnoid spaces (Figs. 4 and 5). The ventricular system, lateral, third and ventricles are enlarged. Microscopically, the cerebral cortex shows patchy loss of nerve cells, arachnoidal thickening, with fibrous elements, much like the brains of cerebral palsy from birth injuries. Other changes are seen in the decrease of nerve fibers, and changes in the myelin sheaths. The atrophic process depends upon the degree of loss of constituent nerve cells and also parallels the degree of intellectual impairment with the resulting behavior disorder. Other conditions described neuropathologically are syndromes of chronic alcoholism, such as Korsakoff's psychosis, alcoholic pellagra, and chronic alcoholic deterioration.

Recently, many observers have shown that the Korsakoff and Wernicke syndromes are really one and the same condition. Both are due to avitaminotic malnutrition, principally thiamin deficiency, occurring secondary to alcoholism.

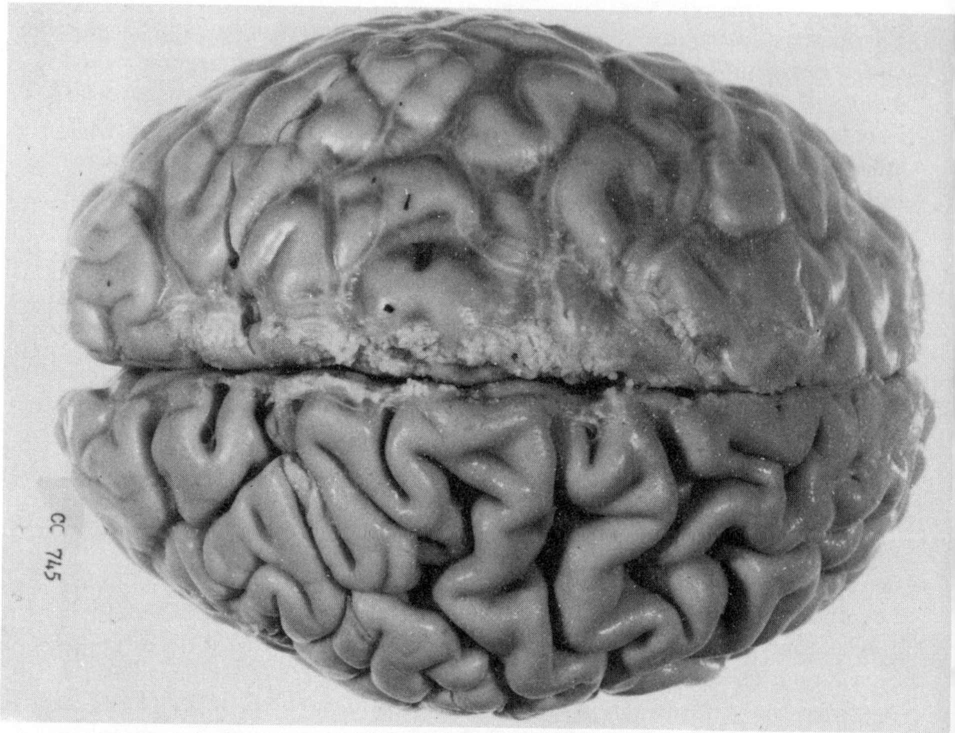

FIG. 2. Alcoholic atrophy of frontal cortex—thickened opaque leptomeninges (from Courville collection).

Clinically, these conditions usually follow one or more episodes of acute delirium. In addition to the midbrain pathology mentioned above, there is some degree of dorsal-lateral convolution frontal lobe atrophy, but not as pronounced as in the chronic alcoholic deterioration.

Alcoholic pellagra has been shown to be due to vitamin B_1 and niacin deficiency. Here there is no gross alteration of the brain, and minimal cortical atrophy occurs. Early proper nutritional treatment is quite effective in this condition. There is usually an associated polyneuropathy and dermatitis.

The postalcoholic dementia or chronic alcoholic deterioration is simply a more advanced progressive stage of alcoholic cortical atrophy which finally produces a vegetative state or death from intercurrent disease. Pathologically, these cases show the above described changes but with more advanced cortical atrophy often associated with progressive ischemia from cerebral arteriosclerosis.

Other neurologic diseases from alcoholism are peripheral neuropathy from vitamin deficiency, possibly associated with cerebral involvement such as alcoholic pellagra or Korsakoff's psychosis, or it may be an isolated entity. This condition is similar to beriberi. Along with alterations in the peripheral nerves there may also be seen anterior horn cells of the spinal cord with other degenerative changes. Here there is a breakdown in the myelin sheaths, with subsequent changes in the axis cylinders, producing the characteristic peripheral neuritis.

Alcoholic cerebellar degeneration is a progressive condition, showing itself by degeneration of the Purkinje cells of cerebellar cortex and fibers, but it is not as common as the cortical atrophy. These atrophic changes are observed grossly and microscopically. Clinically the condition shows itself with progressive ataxia, and in my experience I have found it most difficult to treat and is an irreversible condition when diagnosed. It probably is not the result of vitamin deficiency, as in Korsakoff-Wernicke polyneuropathies.

There is also the rare condition involving the corpus callosm with central necrosis, Marchiafava-Bignami disease, usually seen in Italian wine drinkers. It is associated with either a vitamin deficiency or possibly other exogenous poisonous factors. Arsenic has been attributed as a cause, as it may be used in

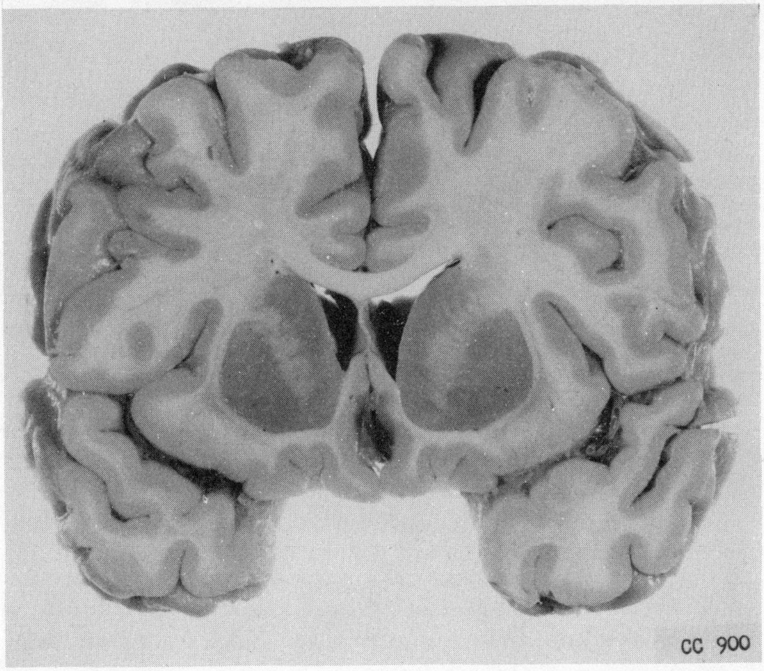

FIG. 3. Alcoholic cortical atrophy—widened sulci—narrowed cortical ribbon.

spraying the grapes in preparation of a wine. Only a few of these cases have been described in the United States.

There are definite spinal cord changes from chronic alcoholism. While rare, these syndromes do occur, such as alterations in the anterior horn cells and posterior columns associated with peripheral neuropathy in chronic alcoholics. There is a clearcut posterior lateral sclerosis syndrome similar to pernicious anemia which is associated with chronic gastritis and anemia, probably from vitamin deficiency. I have also seen spinal cord involvement with alcoholic pellagrous dementia. All of these are due to combinations of alcoholic excess and vitamin nutritional deficiency, principally thiamin and niacin, and usually associated with systemic diseases of the stomach, liver or kidneys.

Fred Lemere and James Smith have attributed alcoholic impotency [8] as due to pathology in the neurogenic reflex arc area of the spinal cord, governing erection, sensory and vasomotor impulses to and from genital organs.

There are other conditions described by Courville that are more the province of neurology than psychiatry, and are related to alcohol and other conditions as

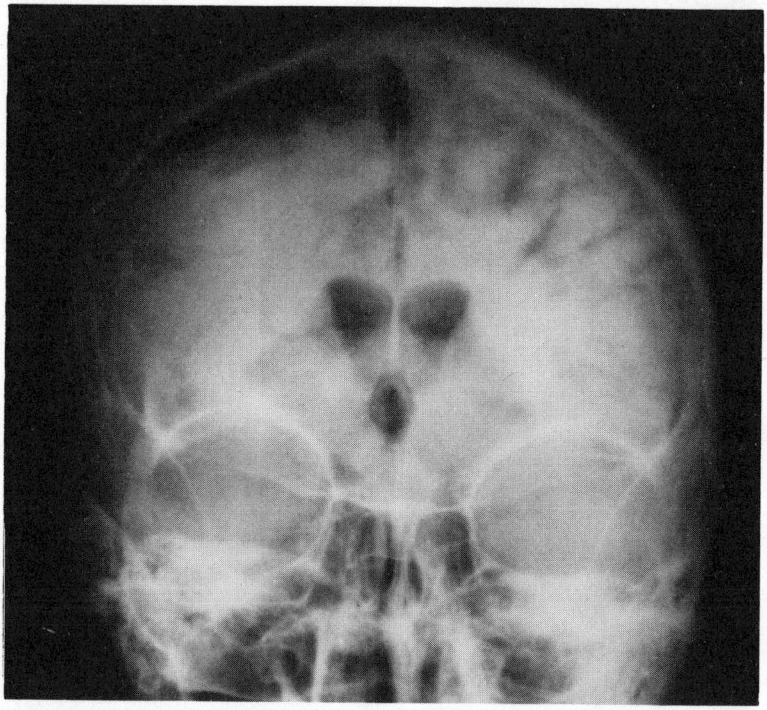

FIG. 4. Early atrophy—widened subarachnoid spaces—ventricular enlargement.

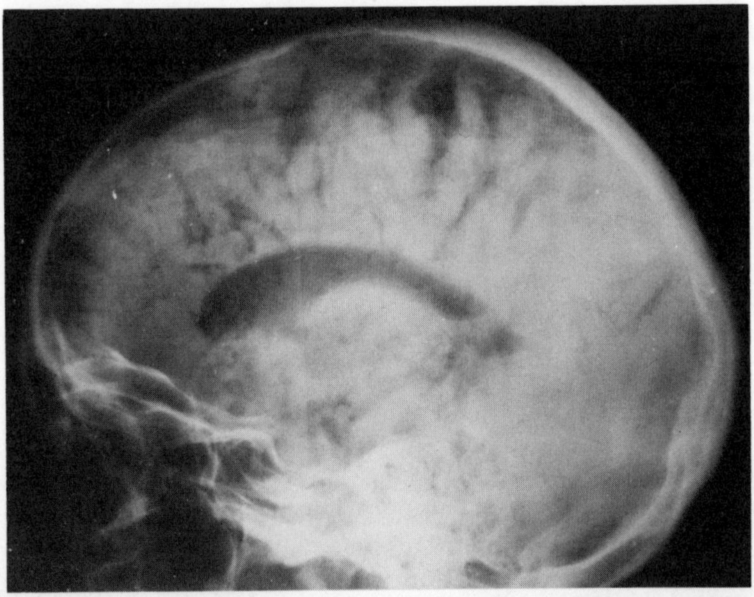

FIG. 5. Cortical atrophy—enlarged lateral ventricle.

follows: alcohol and concussion; traumatic cerebral edema; traumatic meningeal hemorrhage; subdural hematoma.

Other toxemias associated with alcohol are: exogenous poisons such as carbon monoxide, carbon tetrachloride, all the heavy metals, and, most commonly, the associated barbital intoxication from accidental overdose or suicide attempt.

Alcohol and the associated degenerative processes in conjunction with arteriosclerosis produce premature aging and early death in chronic alcoholics.

CHAPTER FOUR

Value of Electroencephalography and Psychological Testing in Alcoholic Brain Disease

Electroencephalography

When we published our study of the value of electroencephalography in alcoholism [6] in 1956, we related our experience in using it as an adjunctive aid in the early diagnosis of alcoholic brain disease. Others have reported extensively on its help in diagnosis and prognosis and explanations of possible mechanisms on what alcohol does to the chronic drinker so far as the brain is concerned. Some have recommended biofeedback training to help alcoholics control drinking, and expressed the idea that periodic EEG examinations might estimate one's tolerance to alcohol. Paul Naitoh [15] reported on the value of electroencephalography in alcoholism in the New York Academy of Medicine symposium, and his conclusions were that it needed further research in all areas in order to determine the true status and value; however, he believed it will be of most value in determining tolerance to alcohol and its relation to the degree of severity of alcoholism, frequency of usage and to susceptibility to addiction because of genetic factors.

We feel that our studies with the clinical application of electroencephalography show it to be of great value in diagnosis and in prognosis of alcoholic brain disease.

From electroencephalographic studies of 758 alcoholic patients (512 male, 246 female) admitted to our psychiatric department in a private general hospital over a period of eight years we found at least a third with abnormal records [6], many of which reversed to normal after sobriety of many months. These cases were either in the intermediate or chronic stages of organic brain disease, in both of which cortical cerebral atrophy was present. If the diagnosis can be made in the intermediate stage, permanent organic deterioration can be prevented. We believe that there are thousands of these cases that go unrecognized. These individuals have reached the phase of the essential pathology of chronic alcoholism, namely compulsive drinking with permanent loss of control over drinking. In cases of slow reversals of the abnormal electroencephalograms we have confirmed the organic basis by psychological testing and in some cases by pneumoencephalography, revealing cortical atrophy. The degree of cortical atrophy usually correlates with the clinical and electroencephalographic findings. Yet there are some chronic cases with severe atrophy that have normal EEG patterns. The same has been seen and treated in cases of advanced paretic dementia [16] and also in some apparently hopeless cases of Korsakoff's disease.

The electroencephalographic findings in general are persistent, mild fast activity 15 to 20 and 4 to 7 per second at times, with paroxysmal slowing and spiking. Fast activity disappears with clinical improvement in acute syndromes. In the acute stage, 37 per cent had abnormal EEG records which reversed to normal but much more slowly. In the chronic stage, 79 per cent had abnormal records, and all of these in both the intermediate and chronic stage showed evidence of organic brain damage (Figs. 6 and 7).

Lafon and co-workers [17] in France compared electroencephalographic and pneumoencephalographic findings in 100 cases of chronic alcoholism. Their pneumograms revealed cerebral atrophy in 78 of the 100 patients, 8 per cent cortical, 40 per cent subcortical, and 48 per cent cortical-subcortical. Of the 100 patients, 80 had abnormal and 20 normal EEG's. In 58 patients, the pneumograms and electroencephalograms could be definitely correlated. In 42 cases there was significant atrophy and yet the EEG's were within normal limits.

In summary, in 758 alcoholic patients admitted to our private general hospital's psychiatric department over the eight-year period we found over one-third with abnormal readings. Many were months in sobriety before reverting to normal. This was the group we studied and classified as the intermediate or chronic stage of alcoholic brain disease. The abnormal EEG's in acute alcoholic syndromes tended to improve to normal within two weeks. The summary of the EEG findings revealed that the most frequently abnormal EEG is fast activity, mostly over the frontal and parietal areas, 14–30 and 4–7 per second, with the fast activity in the acute alcoholic syndrome disappearing with treatment and restoration of normal alpha activity in about two weeks time; however, in most cases there was persistent fast activity, and paroxysmal slowing and spiking in the more chronic cases, some with convulsions and/or delirium. Many of these records persisted for months, and these were the patients who showed severe intellectual impairment or Korsakoff's syndrome.

Computerized tomographic scanning of the brain will largely replace pneumoencephalography and arteriography. We can now see exact areas of localized lesions and all types of cerebral atrophies and hydrocephalus. Its use will clear much of the present confusion in differentiating organic from functional disorders of the brain and aiding in diagnosis and prognosis of alcoholic brain disease.*

James Fox and co-authors† reported cerebral ventricular enlargement in chronic alcoholics by computerized tomography; eight of twelve subjects had

* Twigg, H., Axelbaum, S., Schellinger, D.: Computerized body tomography with ACTA scanner. JAMA 234: 314–317, 1975.

† JAMA 236: 365–368, 1976.

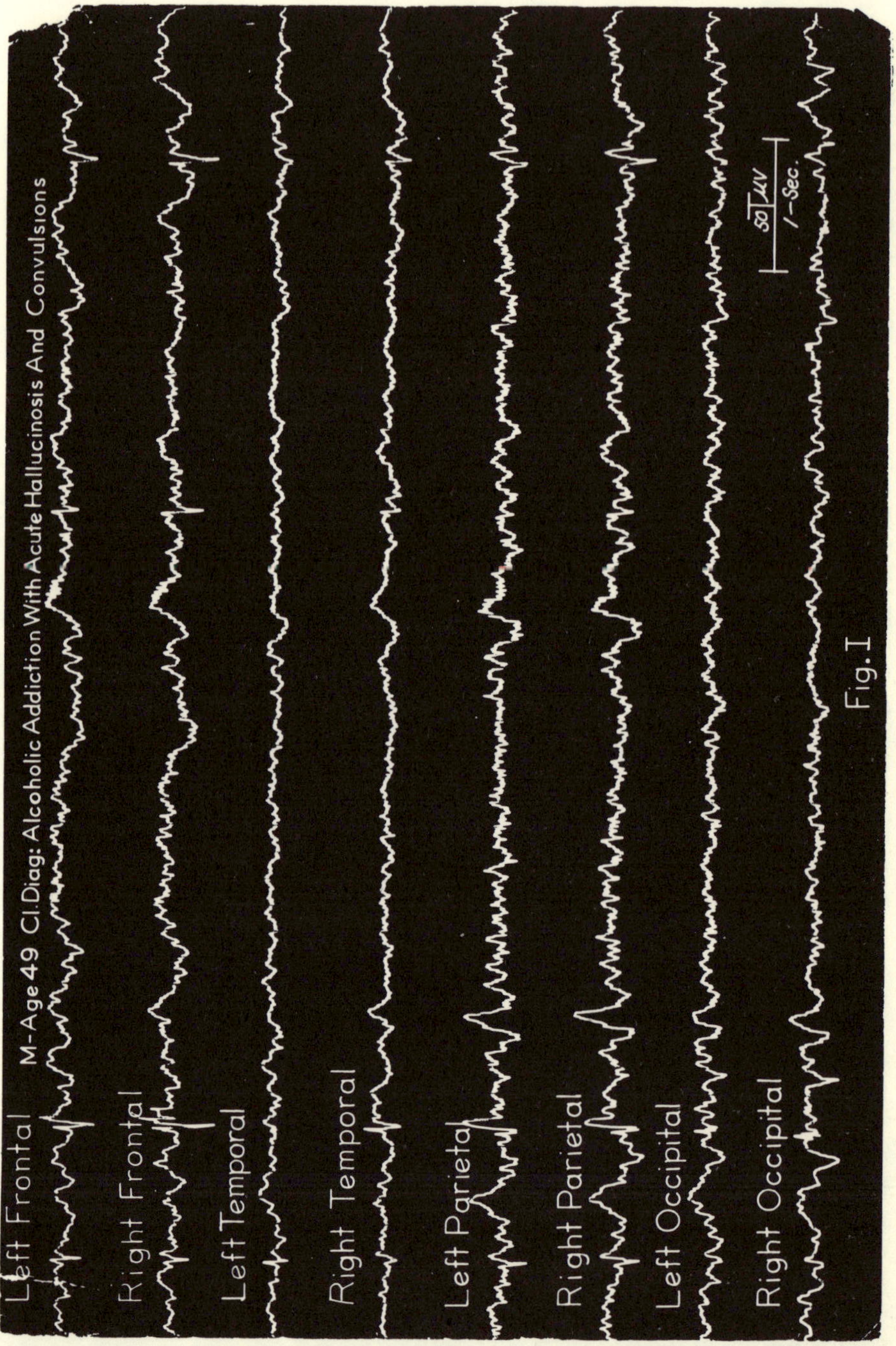

FIG. 6. Electroencephalographic findings.

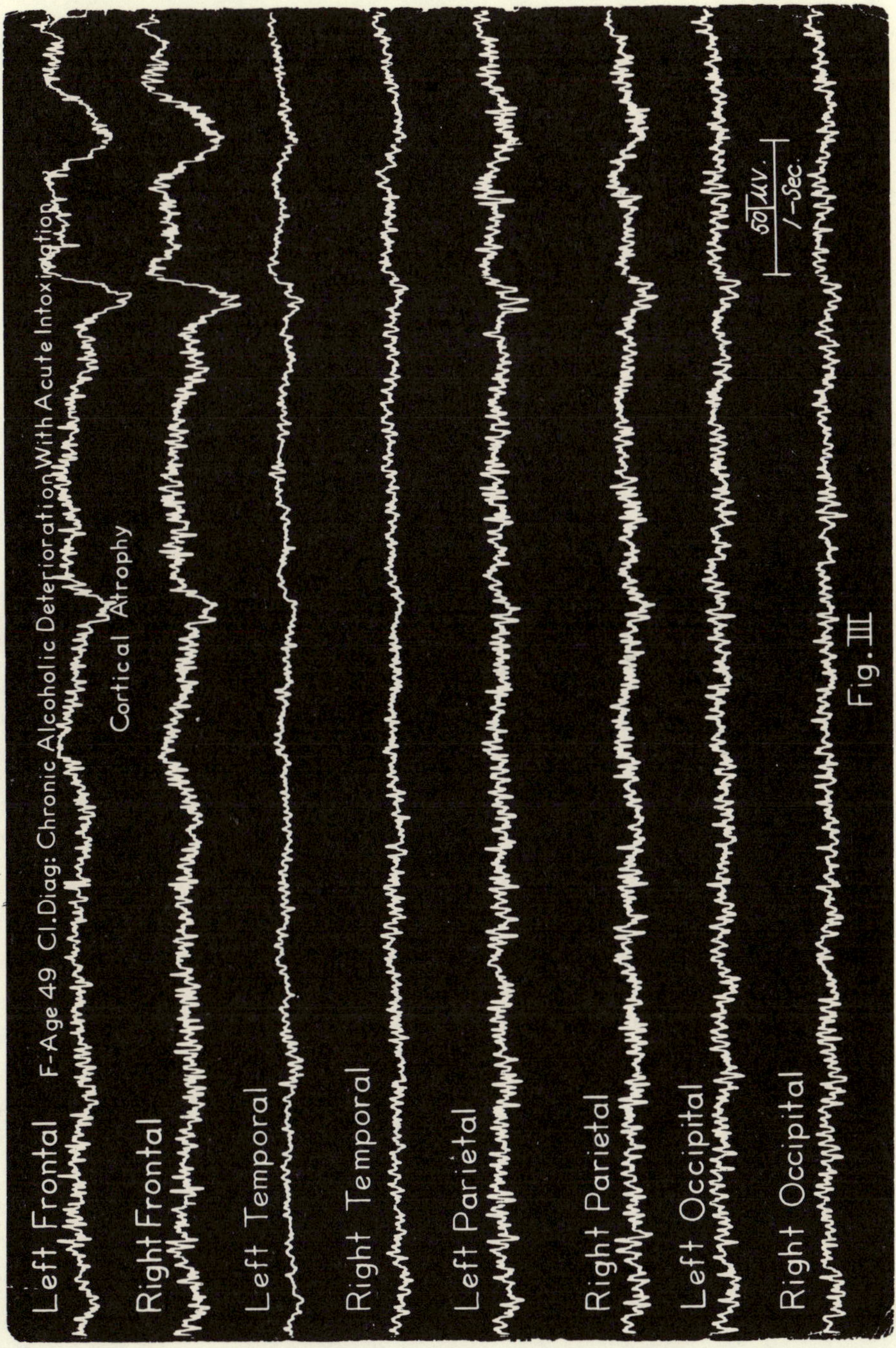

FIG. 7. Electroencephalographic findings.

enlarged ventricles, of which four were markedly enlarged. All had evidence of liver disease and neurologic complications. They reported "simple clinical normal mental status in all patients." They concluded that "enlarged ventricles and possible cerebral atrophy is a prominent symptom of neurologic alcoholism." To me, such reasoning is erroneous; careful psychiatric evaluation would disclose such patients to be in the *intermediate stage of alcoholic brain disease.* The direct and indirect effects of alcohol upon the cerebral cortex produce the atrophy, and the neurologic disorders are concomitants of alcoholic brain disease.

*Psychological Testing**

Research Findings

In recent years, there has been an upsurge in research on the psychological effects of alcoholism. In a comprehensive review, Tarter [18] summarizes observations of intellectual functioning in alcoholics. Within the group of studies cited, surprisingly little cognitive impairment was found. Intelligence, as measured by standardized tests, was not globally impaired. However, there was a consistent trend toward greater sparing of verbal than visuomotor skills. Overlearned skills, those that are used frequently, showed greater resistance to deterioration than those practiced less often. In alcoholics, there can be a striking contrast between the level of skill in practiced habits and that when new problems are approached.

There also were some findings of impaired voluntary motor activity. Frequent causes appeared to be such correlates of alcoholism as peripheral neuropathy, muscle atrophy and cerebellar degeneration. Both speed and dexterity of movement were affected. When these purely motor deficiencies were taken into account, there appeared to be little or no reduction of eye-hand coordination. That is, eye-hand coordination was essentially intact, but the efficiency of the hand itself was affected. Deficits also appeared in the comprehension of space. Copies of drawings or constructions showed internal distortions. There was impairment of the ability to maintain constant bearings on the true vertical and true horizontal. This applied to the sense of body position as well as the orientation of external objects. In the most literal sense, the subjects were "tipsy."

* This section on *Psychological Testing* is by Nancy V. Van Couvering, Ph.D., Director, Clinical Neuropsychology Program, Veterans Administration Hospital, Martinez, California.

Other higher functions were affected. Verbal memory was spared, but the learning of new material was impaired. Reasoning processes showed deficits commonly associated with frontal lobe dysfunction. Compared to normals, alcoholics were more: (1) concrete (literal minded), (2) rigid (unable to change from one mental set to the next), (3) unable to recognize and/or correct errors in their own performance, and (4) perseverative (unable to extinguish a behavior sequence after engaging in it).

Studies of personality continue to indicate that there is not a unique personality that is prone to alcoholism. Some personality types show a greater vulnerability, however. Personality disorders seem especially prone to include alcoholism among their other behavioral excesses (Dahlstrom [19]).

Clinical Manifestations in Psychological Testing

Psychological testing is useful in clarifying the status of an alcoholic, because an ongoing drinking problem is often reflected there before the appearance of physical stigmata. There are four areas where measurable changes occur in psychological functioning: (1) memory, (2) perceptual-motor skills, (3) reasoning and abstract thinking (verbal and perceptual), and (4) motivational-emotional functioning, but there is no such thing as a specific alcoholic mentality. These changes are in reference to pre-morbid baselines for the individual, and detected by deflections from residual baselines obtained from the individual.

Memory can be affected by alcohol in several ways, and the memory defects appear in all levels of voluntary behavior. Clinicians are familiar with the confabulations and forgetfulness accompanying Korsakoff's dementia. In earlier alcoholic brain disease there are more subtle manifestations of memory loss. These milder memory lapses have a distinctive quality which differentiates alcoholics from psychotics or other organics. Although most non-alcoholics with memory problems are aware of them, alcoholics seem unaware of the magnitude of the deficit. Many show a generalized defect in short-term memory, often with mild perseverative or confabulatory tendencies which may be evident only on structured tests.

When alcoholics confabulate, it is as if they have lost the templates which make it possible to identify correct memories. Lacking this capacity, one "memory" apparently seems as reasonable as the next. Therefore, the most plausible or most familiar item is misidentified as correct. Errors created by this process may be severe in extent, but the *content* of the errors is not likely to be bizarre or idiosyncratic. For example, a fasting patient may report having eaten a hearty breakfast of bacon and eggs. The mildness of these confabulations, combined with the person's own lack of awareness, sometimes allows such lapses to pass unnoticed by the interviewer. In alcoholic perseveration, responses are repeated when no longer appropriate. For example, in verbal learning tasks, a word once learned may be given in response to later questions, or even during later tests.

Perceptual-motor skills show characteristic defects. In graphic tasks, the person may see (and draw) double. Line quality is heavy and tremulous at the same time. (In other conditions, if tremulousness is present the line quality usually is light and spidery.) Line junctions are crude, and angles are blunted. Although the person may copy from a model accurately, productions from memory often err in being oversimplified, or perseveration may occur. For example, the person may reproduce a perspective drawing of a cube from memory. In later tasks of the same type, the cube may reappear, very likely in simplified form, perhaps now as a square.

In alcoholics who are drinking, capacities for reasoning and abstraction are reduced. Interpretations become literal, so that "Strike while the iron is hot" translates as "Something to do with bending metal?," or, "One swallow doesn't make a summer" becomes "You mean a bird or a drink?", or, "No, it takes a whole bottle to make it seem like summer." Effects of a more subtle nature can appear in verbal analogies or vocabulary definitions. Responses are given in terms of functions or attributes, instead of the higher categories to which the item belongs. For instance, on the WAIS [20], the answer to the "table-chair" analogy might be "legs" or "to eat on," instead of "furniture." Similar effects appear in definitions of words, so that "penny" is "round" instead of "coin." Not infrequently, an alcoholic will give a concrete response first and then work up to a more abstract one.

When a person is drinking, perceptual reasoning often is affected. On tasks such as block designs, errors are less likely to stem from perceptual confusion than an inability to organize the pattern elements. Simple clues are overlooked, such as the fact that symmetrical patterns must have the same number of blocks on each side. When hints are given at this level, there may be no further difficulty in solving that problem, but little generalization to the next.

The quality of the effect of alcohol on cognitive skills is fairly consistent across individuals. The severity appears to be at least in part a function of the length of time since the person's last drink. Test effects tend to persist for some time after the physical findings are clear. It is not unusual for some of the stigmata to be recorded after six weeks' abstinence. A mild memory deficit may linger for several months after that. Eventually, if the person continues to drink, the effects can become chronic. Page and Linden [21] reported persistent organic dysfunction in long-term drinkers. Whether this is a direct or secondary effect of alcohol is a point of contention. Whatever the cause, it is possible to identify people with substantial histories of alcoholism by their tendencies toward perceptual and verbal concreteness, reduced fine motor control and forgetfulness.

Withdrawal Effects

Psychiatric changes also are tied to recency of drinking, except in cases of advanced mental deterioration. In heavy drinkers, withdrawal effects can be expected after about 24 hours of abstinence. The person becomes irritable, hypervigilant and tremulous. Alcoholics refer to this condition as "the whips and shakes." The person feels weak, and becomes weaker and more shaky with exertion. This condition usually lasts from 10 to 14 days. During this period, alcoholics are not enthusiastic about psychological testing.

When they do cooperate, some characteristic indicators appear in the findings. The MMPI [22] personality profile shows high paired peaks on Scale 2 (Depression) and Scale 8 (Schizophrenia), in a pattern typical for organic conditions (Dahlstrom [19]). Alcoholics tend to be unique in showing an elevation of Scale 7 (Psychasthenia) that approaches or exceeds that of Scale 8. The remaining clinical scales give some indication of the premorbid personality structure, and the over-all pattern indicates that this individual is suffering from depression, loss of mental control and anxiety.

On the WAIS, the Verbal IQ is higher than the Performance IQ, but the difference is not necessarily extreme (Ryan [23]). The Factor III subtests, Arithmetic, Digit Span and Digit Symbol, show a stair-step progression downward, with Digit Symbol being the lowest in the profile. This pattern is typical for many organics (Denerll [24]), and is an indicator of distractibility/short-term memory deficit. The Similarities subtest tends to be depressed. On the Wechsler Memory Scale [25], there may be mild confabulation in the errors on the Logical Memory subtest and distortions on the Visual Recall subtest. Tremulousness and coarse line quality appear in graphic productions.

In alcoholic hallucinosis, the pattern is much more suggestive of organicity than schizophrenia. Hallucinations are more visual than auditory, and sometimes involve other sensory modalities. The content may include ideas of persecution, but the grandiosity and ideas of reference found in schizophrenics are not present. Often, the alcoholic can locate the hallucinated object in space. There is not the concern about etiology seen in non-alcoholics, as a rule. This relative lack of concern extends to "blackouts" (amnestic episodes) and withdrawal seizures. Although the MMPI shows elevations on Scales F and 8, the person does not appear thought-disordered either clinically or on the Rorschach [26]. After three or four days of withdrawal, the person may go into delirium. This severe medical condition includes profound psychological involvement, but psychological testing is not indicated at this time.

Effects of Nutritional Deficiencies

In addition to the withdrawal syndromes noted above, there are other conditions resulting from nutritional deficiency. The most familiar is Wernicke's—Korsakoff's disease. This may (or may not) be accompanied by peripheral neuropathy and/or cerebellar degeneration, or the latter may appear independently.

The ocular disturbances of Wernicke's syndrome preclude using psychological tests requiring the person to fill out machine-scored answer sheets, such as the MMPI group forms, although the box form may be used. The person experiences difficulty trying to grasp visual stimuli composed only of lines, without texturally differentiated internal masses, such as the Picture Arrangement subtest of the WAIS. Perceptual distortions (simplification, perseveration) accompany the visual ones.

In Wernicke's syndrome the mental state is one of anxiety and depressed confusion. Little conversation is volunteered. If an MMPI is obtained at this point, the profile usually is quite flat, hovering around 50 (T + K), possibly with slight elevations on Scales 2 and/or 8. The Rorschach protocol often is grossly organic, with an impoverished global approach, failures and perseverated content (dead moths, decayed leaves with centerline stems, etc.).

There is disorientation which includes the identity of other persons. Although these misidentifications are colorful, they usually make sense in terms of the person's history. For example, a treatment room may be mistaken for part of a jail or rescue mission, or physicians and nurses for relatives or drinking buddies. Such confabulations are part of a generalized memory defect which includes gaps in the person's past history and makes the acquisition of new learning almost impossible.

This amnestic-confabulatory condition is captured admirably by the Wechsler Memory Scale (Forms I and II). The Memory Quotient (MQ) yielded by this test is less informative than the quality of errors in performance. In the errors, new content of a non-bizarre nature appears. For example, in the Logical Memory subtest, "Anna Thompson of South Boston" may become "Anna Jones of South Dakota." Even though the ensuing story bears little resemblance to the model, it often shows internal consistency. Or, on the Paired Associates subtest, errors of a high-probability type appear so that "School-Grocery" may become "School-Books."

In Korsakoff's syndrome, there are mild to moderate perceptual distortions and visual concreteness. There also is a tendency toward verbal concreteness and cognitive rigidity. Most outstandingly, there is a profound defect of memory. Confabulation may occur, but not necessarily. Overlearned skills are spared, such as those measured by the WAIS Vocabulary and Comprehension subtests. However, there is retrograde amnesia, so that prior events are forgotten. New learning is acquired with difficulty and tends to decay rapidly. The memory deficit leaves the person vulnerable to confusion and consequent fearfulness, unless living in sheltered surroundings. Another result can be garrulousness, because the individual forgets the topic and rambles until diverted.

In psychological testing, results show mild to moderate impairment, with greater sparing of verbal than performance skills. There is a marked memory defect. Often, there is depression in part reactive to loss of competence. Ryan [23] suggests that the memory problem may not be one of storage, but of inefficient mnemonic strategies. If, on the test findings, verbal and performance deficits prove to be of comparable severity, and especially if there is a significant verbal component in a picture of spotty deficits, this is suggestive of cortical atrophy.

With cerebellar degeneration, the longer a continuous unidirectional movement is sustained, such as reaching slowly for something, the more coarse the directional control becomes. Aside from the tremulousness, which reduces speed and control in performance tasks, there is no direct representation of this condition in psychological test results. Peripheral neuropathy also has a limited effect on testing, but it can confound the unwary interpreter. It can produce stocking and glove anesthesias, which should not be mistaken for hysterical manifestations. Neuropathy can interfere in tests requiring tactile and sensory acuity, such as the Purdue Pegboard [27] and parts of the Halstead-Reitan battery [28].

Implications for Counseling

It is important to recognize with cerebral involvement that attitudinal and emotional metacommunications may be all that get through to the person. Poor memory, coupled with a tendency toward literal-mindedness, make it difficult for the person to follow a logical argument, let alone remember the reasons for not drinking when needed. It is certain that the counselor who expects a brain-damaged alcoholic to stop drinking solely through sweet reason or guided insight is going to have a long wait. The success of the approach developed by Alcoholics Anonymous undoubtedly is due to the fact that their appeal is not based on logic alone. Alcoholics are not all alike, though brain disease may create similarities in psychological functions. Treatment must be individually planned to be effective. The results of clinical evaluation, personality changes, and history from informants provide data for assessing the degree of cerebral functioning. Electroencephalography and psychological testing can help confirm the clinical diagnosis and prognosis, and guide appropriate treatment.

CHAPTER FIVE

Associated Systemic Diseases; Morbidity and Mortality; Medicolegal Problems in Alcoholism and Industry

While this monograph is primarily a review of the knowledge of the effects of alcohol on the nervous system, it seems appropriate to discuss the highlights of associated systemic diseases, particularly those that might affect the brain. Also a brief discussion of morbidity and mortality of chronic alcoholism seems to belong in this review. All of the following systemic complications are common in alcoholic brain disease. They have to be treated along with alcoholic brain damage in rehabilitation.

Stomach: In acute alcoholism there is produced congestion, hemorrhages with increased mucous and varying degrees of ulceration, depending upon the amount of alcohol ingested. In chronic alcoholism the commonest disorder is gastritis with atrophy of the mucosa and associated achlohydria. This is usually associated with anemia and spinal cord changes similar to those seen in pernicious anemia; posterior lateral column degeneration can occur.

Liver: In acute alcoholism there is a cloudy swelling of liver cells, while in chronic alcoholism there is fatty infiltration that leads to cirrhosis and often hemorrhages resulting from esophageal varices. Liver insufficiency leading to cardiac death can occur, and 64 per cent of the cases of delirium tremens show associated fatty or cirrhotic livers. Alcohol causes gastrointestinal disorders due to its irritating action upon mucous membranes, producing gastritis, enteritis, pancreatitis and nutritional deficiencies.

Pancreas: Alcoholism has been shown to be responsible for about 50 per cent of chronic pancreatitis and 68 per cent of the acute attacks of pancreatitis are precipitated by bouts with alcohol. About 20 per cent of those who die of or develop chronic relapsing pancreatic disease have a history of alcoholism. In acute alcoholism deaths 25% have acute pancreatitis.

Heart and Circulation: Specific cardiac disorders occur from heavy chronic drinking. Cardiac myopathy similar to arteriosclerotic heart disease may occur. Myocardosis and cardiac failure come from heavy beer drinking. Both of these entities are different from beri-beri heart disease from vitamin B deficiency. Summarizing essential information about cardiomyopathies, it is estimated that there are about 10,000 alcoholic adults who have clinical cardiomyopathy, making it one of the most frequent of the cardiomuscular diseases. The prognosis is grave and abstinence from alcohol is a must for recovery. "Any sign of cardiac dysfunction not otherwise explained in a person consuming moderate to large amounts of alcohol warrants discontinuance of alcohol, since advanced stages may not be reversible."* Alcohol probably should be discouraged in patients with coronary artery disease.

Accidents and Suicides Associated with Alcoholism

Many studies show that over 50 per cent of highway fatalities, totaling over 25,000 yearly, show high alcohol blood levels in the drivers. 20,000 fatalities from other alcohol-related accidents occur annually.

In completed suicides, studies show that from one-third to one-half had high alcohol blood levels; the same applied in 40 to 50 per cent of unsuccessful attempts. More than 15,000 alcohol-related suicides and homicides occur annually.

If we could evaluate all the direct and indirect causes of death in which alcohol is involved we could put alcoholism as the third cause of death. Government vital statistics do not reveal these facts. For instance, the official statistics of 1964 listed deaths from alcoholism at only 11,000. Just as with suicide mortality figures, these are highly misleading. There is a reluctance to certify alcoholism as a cause of death. The Metropolitan Life Insurance Company states that it is fairly certain that the greater proportion of cirrhosis of the liver is alcohol-associated and in some cities is listed as the fifth cause of death. We made a study of all alcohol-related deaths and coroners' findings (not published) and concluded that over 100,000 deaths occur annually from alcoholism.

Alcohol-related deaths are increasing. Life insurance companies estimate that longevity is curtailed ten to twelve years in chronic alcoholics. Insurance underwriters estimate that among people with a history of alcoholism, the death rate is three times higher than among non-drinkers.

Another serious aspect of chronic alcoholism is the effect of alcohol upon the morphogenesis in babies of chronic alcoholic women. Jones and colleagues at Washington School of Medicine have reported a series of cases followed for seven years. They studied particularly the abnormalities of CNS function. They found a 17 per cent perinatal mortality rate compared with 2 per cent for the control group, and 43 per cent had an adverse outcome in the pregnancies: diminished head circumference, deficient intellectual performance with low

* Parker, B. M.: The effects of alcohol on the heart. JAMA 28: 741–742, 1974.

I.Q.'s as tested at seven years, and other fetal alcoholic syndromes such as bone joint and cardiac anomalies.

Medicolegal Problems in Alcoholism

George N. Thompson [29] has given a very comprehensive discussion of a problem he calls acute pathologic alcoholic intoxication and its medicolegal implications. A summary of his formulation is as follows. Clinically, pathologic alcoholic intoxication has become probably the most important alcoholic disorder that comes to the attention of administrators of the law. Although this disorder is less common than several other alcoholic mental disorders, its importance legally is due to the fact that crimes of extreme violence are often committed while the individual is in this state. Homicide is a not infrequent result of an attack of this disease, and usually the initial criminal charge is that of murder. These crimes result from the clinical characteristics of the disorder.

The disease occurs usually in previously brain-injured individuals or those who have had a brain disease or other organic abnormality. Thompson also states that he feels that it can derive from alcoholic brain damage in certain individuals. The disease or traumatic process is usually in the frontal or temporal lobes or their connections with the thalamus. The afflicted individual exhibits abnormal behavior responses to relatively small amounts of alcohol, amounts which would normally have only minor effects on the average person. Total or partial amnesia follows. During the period of amnesia the afflicted individual carries out behavior that is automatic. To the unaware observer, the behavior may appear consciously motivated. In this and almost all other respects, Thompson believes that acute pathologic alcoholic intoxication and psychomotor epilepsy are essentially the same disease. He states that alcohol per se may be the primary cause of the disorder, and if sufficient alcoholic brain deterioration occurs in the critical tracts of the brain, the disorder will appear, and thus trauma is not the only cause. Other neuropathologic lesions also may be factors. The main criterion of the disease is usually electroencephalographic evidence. The electroencephalogram does not make the diagnosis, it merely confirms it, or aids in suspicious cases. Furthermore, therapeutic amounts of alcoholic intake may reproduce an attack. The characteristic electroencephalographic abnormalities are three: (1) localized spiking, usually temporal or frontal lobe; (2) high-voltage slow wave bursts, also temporal and frontal, 2–6 cycle per second; (3) spike and slow wave mixtures, again in localized bursts.

Thompson reported a number of cases, including their trial in court. He summarizes by stating that acute alcoholic pathologic intoxication is a most important alcoholic mental disorder in legal medicine and with every legal presentation can be shown to be "legal insanity." The electroencephalogram, while not essential to the diagnosis, is confirmatory and legal proof and is sometimes required by courts of law. He recommends that individuals with this disorder should be required to register with local health departments, undergo periodic examinations and remain under medical treatment throughout their lives, and that this control should be required by law.

Marinacci [30] reported reproducing psychomotor encephalographic patterns in patients suspected of having suffered from pathologic intoxication with small amounts of alcohol. In one series of sixty patients he found twelve who had paroxysmal wave patterns after ingestion of small amounts of alcohol. We, too,* have found that small amounts of alcohol will produce seizure patterns in some cases of latent psychomotor epilepsy and have used this technic as evidence in court cases upon murders similar to those described by Thompson. In my experience, jurists and juries have not been willing to accept this evidence as legal insanity and have convicted the accused as murderers.

Another important medicolegal problem with which I have been involved a number of times is the question of incompetency in brain damaged alcoholics. Many alcoholics in high positions with great responsibility can jeopardize an industry through their poor judgment [31]. In other cases, they make out wills cutting out their rightful heirs and leave estates to individuals who supply them with alcohol. Family members should get a psychiatric evaluation of such alcoholics to protect their legitimate interests, in case of death. This is often not easy to do without voluntary cooperation from the patient. I have witnessed a number of deplorable situations where undeserving individuals have been able to influence the sick alcoholic to cut out his rightful heirs by undue influence, encouraging ingestion of alcohol or fostering paranoid delusions. Brain damage in the alcoholic opens the door to such connivings. A recent example was the case of a 74 year old divorced man, a severe alcoholic for many years, in and out of hospitals and residence homes for a period of five years with chronic polyneuropathy, liver disease, repeated gastrointestinal hemorrhages and subject to seizures and delirium. He left his considerable estate to a female employee who had continued to supply him with alcohol and had taken over his business and family affairs. He felt his children were conspiring against him and cut them out of his will, conveying his money and property to his employee. After his death, the son and daughter started suit to set aside the will on the basis of incompetency. The hospital records, carefully evaluated, left no doubt of the patient's intellectual impairment, with marked personality changes. Just as the case was about to be tried, a cash settlement was made. I

* Bennett, A. E.: Mental disorders with temporal lobe epilepsy. Dis. Nerv. Syst. 26: 275–279, 1965.

have been consulted on several similar cases but know of none that have been tried in the courts to settle the issue of mental incompetence in brain damaged alcoholics in will cases.

The Effects of Alcoholism upon Brain Function and Its Relation to Industry

Leaders in progressive companies realize that alcoholic problems in industry are both prevalent and costly. In the past, these problems have been largely ignored or treated by censure, without offering the victims rehabilitation. Employers who recognize early symptoms of alcoholism in employees can help them before their jobs are jeopardized and get real dividends while saving their investment in the employee. There are a number of companies who have well established rehabilitation programs and appreciate their value. Those who ignore or fail to understand the disease concept of alcoholism, and simply fire the employee rather than encourage treatment, need enlightment on how to salvage a useful employee and save money. Some good alcoholism industry programs report that 80% are rehabilitated.

A recent American Medical Association editorial estimates that 4–5 per cent of the employee population is involved in problem drinking and secondary results from absenteeism or decreased work production cost industry 4 billion dollars annually. Chafetz, of the National Institute on Alcoholism, estimates 10% of the nation's work force is involved, at a total cost to the national economy of 15 billion dollars a year in lost time and other effects.

What are some of the signs pointing to a possible alcoholic problem that supervisors should watch for in an employee?

1. *Hangover absences.* Frequent absences from work, either during the week or especially after paydays or holidays, may be a sign of an alcoholic problem. Such workers often give odd or improbable excuses for their absenteeism or they claim to be suffering from colds, flu, stomach trouble or other minor illnesses. Frequently, their excuses are irrational, due to alcoholic thinking, and lying is part of their defense and cover-up.

2. *Injuries on the job.* Alcoholics have three times as many accidents as normal persons because of poor judgment, faulty coordination or tremulousness resulting from drinking.

3. *Significant drop in work efficiency.* Alcoholics tend to work in spurts or to be overly careful to avoid accidents, thus wasting time.

4. *Any evidence of intoxication during working hours or odor of alcohol on the employee's breath.*

5. *Changes in personality.* Persons with a drinking problem often display shifting moods (e.g., from affability to sensitiveness to criticism of their drinking, or increased suspiciousness shown by resentfulness or sarcasm).

6. *Problems away from work.* The problem drinker often gets himself into domestic, financial or community difficulties. If these problems coincide with psychological or physical evidence of drinking, they are indications of a problem drinker.

7. *Changes in drinking patterns.* Lack of control over drinking—e.g., drinking more than the others, or between rounds, when drinking with fellow employees after working hours, or being unable to stop drinking—are important danger signals indicative of a compulsive alcoholic.

If any of these evidences of an alcoholic problem are present, it is a supervisor's responsibility to have a frank talk with the employee. The worker should be told about his poor work performance, absenteeism or other factors which indicate a drinking problem. He should not be accused of being an alcoholic but told that a problem with alcohol is suspected. If the employee agrees, a treatment program should be discussed. If he does not agree, he may be given the responsibility of improving his job performance; however, if this does not improve in one month, he may have to be pressured into seeking help or referred to the company medical department, which may have to decide whether job separation is necessary to get positive action toward treatment.

Firm company policies must be based on the understanding that alcoholism is a health problem which can be treated; that the company will aid in proper treatment; that the company will give the employee every opportunity to obtain treatment, but that job termination will occur if there is no improvement. By constructive coercion, obtaining recognition from the employee that he has a drinking problem and the understanding that he will lose his job if drinking is not controlled, complete motivation can usually be obtained.

The understanding of alcoholism's effect upon brain function is of extreme importance to all leaders of industry. Alcoholics with brain damage occupying important positions can be extremely costly to management because of progressive intellectual deterioration. These cases must be recognized as early as possible by medical examiners and entered into rehabilitation programs and treated for organic features of brain damage. Many can be salvaged, while those with advanced irreversible disease should be recognized and removed from positions of responsibility.

Many companies have alcohol control programs for the estimated five million alcoholics still working. Sixty of the four hundred largest corporations have become involved. General Motors Corporation has alcoholism committees in all plants. They show a 50 per cent cut in lost man hours, 30 per cent drop in sickness and accident benefits, 56 per cent drop in absenteeism, and 60 to 80 per cent reduction in grievances filed, disciplinary problems and job-related accidents. By using constructive coercion, supervisors and physicians were able to motivate and rehabilitate 70% of those enrolled in the programs. By treating alcoholism as a disease and using trained counselors, the workers were given a choice of treatment or losing their job. They receive sick leave and medical benefits. Unions are also cooperating. Patients are referred to A.A., V.A hospitals, mental hospitals or private agencies for definitive treatment.

Another medicolegal problem that is being badly mishandled for society's protection is the drinking driver. Despite increasingly strict laws, including mandatory alcohol testing, the drunken driver continues to cause most of our highway accidents. Often, by paying for expensive lawyer services, he can escape punishment. Some judges have alcoholic problems themselves and are inclined to leniency. Only a few enlightened lawyers understand alcoholism as a disease, or the effects of alcohol in producing brain damage. What is needed is orientation of the judiciary toward treatment instead of punishment, and coercive referral of all convicted drivers into a comprehensive treatment program with revoking of driving license until a physician certifies that the patient has had sustained sobriety for one year. After that, if he is competent to return to driving he should be continued on periodic check-ups to insure that he is not relapsed. Many of my brain-damaged alcoholic patients have been able to keep their drivers license by paying high legal fees.

While I am constantly being asked to pass on the safety of some patient as to his competence to drive a motor vehicle after being under hospital treatment for an emotional disorder, I've never been asked by the highway motor vehicle department for an opinion on an alcoholic under my treatment who has been seriously ill from chronic alcoholism. A few enlightened judges are placing drinking drivers on probation, provided they seek help, with very effective results. Much more publicity about these programs is needed. All applicants for licenses or renewals should be thoroughly investigated as to problems with alcohol before licenses are issued.

Epileptics are under strict surveillance even if well controlled by medication. These periodic reports are necessary but nowhere near as important as getting the alcohol-involved driver off our highways. Current efforts cost the taxpayer large amounts of money without being really effective. State laws need overhauling, with expert guidance from informed people to make the laws affecting drunk drivers serve a useful purpose, not only for sick alcoholics themselves but for the protection of others on our highways. Until this is done, the needless carnage will continue and probably grow worse.

CHAPTER SIX

Psychiatric Alcoholic Brain Disorders

The Making of an Alcoholic

In all kinds of alcoholics the cause is too much alcohol. The commonest type is the result of an addictive drug upon an unstable, emotionally immature person. When a man desires alcohol more than he loves his family, work, or social standing, he has become an addictive alcoholic. He now lives for alcohol; alcohol controls his life. This is mental illness, a compulsive addictive disorder.

Generally, he uses alcohol to evade obligations or escape from an intolerable situation. As an anesthetic, it dulls his sensibilities by its depressing action, thereby relieving his feelings of inadequacy.

Drinking Patterns Leading to Addiction

How is an alcoholic made? The borderlines between the so-called social drinker, the problem drinker, and the chronic alcoholic are far from clearcut. The average alcoholic develops as follows: The early stage is social drinking, in which he drinks alcohol like other beverages, for social rather than for anesthetic effects. After three to four years of such drinking, certain individuals start to be compulsive, dependent drinkers. They gradually increase the amount of alcohol, taking doubles instead of singles to relieve anxiety and reduce frustration or resentment, and sneaking extras at cocktail parties. They rely more and more upon alcohol as they find they cannot relax without it. In the meantime, their tolerance increases; they take more and more to meet individual needs until they become confirmed heavy drinkers.

After a period of heavy drinking (on the average, about ten years), they become uncontrolled drinkers. Some individuals get to this stage within a few years. Women alcoholics may reach this stage faster because of secretive drinking and erratic eating, with poor nutrition. Now the occasional "pass-outs" or blackouts begin—temporary periods of amnesia from the drinking events. While there is no loss of consciousness, still the victim can recall little of what happened. He may, for example, drive away, register at a motel, and upon awakening cannot recollect how he got there. He may do very dramatic things, such as participating in a violent crime, much as in an epileptic episode. These symptoms are the first definite warnings of early brain damage, with loss of control. If the individual can be made to see the danger of these states, he may become frightened and seek help.

The person now becomes concerned over his source of supply and begins to protect it, ensuring enough for weekends, when he gets drunk. Later on, he drinks every evening. Evening drinking gradually extends into daytime drinking, with drinking on the job and before breakfast to cure the hangover. He hides bottles or other containers from the family, especially his spouse. Ashamed of his drinking, he tends to skip meals, to drop his interests and hobbies, replacing them more and more with alcoholic indulgence.

Later Stages

Because of the development of partial tolerance, the alcoholic has to drink more and more to get drunk. In the absence of beverage alcohol, he resorts to such non-beverage alcohol as vanilla extract or shaving lotion. The alcoholic "binges" extend from weekends to several days, then to several weeks. In the blackouts he becomes more confused. The definite physical symptoms that usually appear may be ushered in by convulsions or delirium tremens, alcoholic tremors, insomnia, general physical decline, gastritis with morning vomiting, and symptoms of liver disease. His first hospital experience may follow. Some persons even go through treatment for these complications without the true cause being uncovered, because the patient denies or conceals it from the physician, or the physician is not sufficiently alert to look for it, especially in secretive female alcoholics.

Serious social aspects also come into the picture. The marriage is threatened; children avoid their parents and are ashamed to bring playmates home. Absenteeism from work finally leads to loss of the job and other financial losses, e.g., waste of money at bars or in bad business ventures. At this point the individual may lose all his social contacts and seek fellow alcoholics at bars or get into trouble with the law, often on drunk-driving charges. More fortunately, he may break down physically and land in the hospital. These signs of deterioration have been obvious for a long time to everyone but the patient.

By this time, the patient has usually tried manifold ways to control excessive drinking. He sets up certain goals. For example, he won't drink alone or will take only two and quit, or only drink beer, or he may go "on the wagon" for a time. But he slips repeatedly and always ends up in compulsive drinking, unless he faces up to the fact that he has to quit, gains the motivation and mental discipline never ever to drink again, accepting total abstinence as the only cure for chronic alcoholism.

Usually, then, he avoids serious thinking. He can't face giving up completely or substitute anything else for alcohol. He still imagines that he can drink in a controlled fashion. He manufactures all sorts of alibis and rationalizations (Alcoholics Anonymous calls them "alcoholic thinking") to account for his mistakes and his symptoms of ill health. He steadily denies that these symptoms could be the result of his alcoholism and believes he has fooled others by his denials and lies.

After sustained excessive drinking, organic factors arise from alcoholic brain damage and contribute to the loss of control of drinking. Judgment and emotional centers for self-control are impaired, and these changes are often considered to be neurotic. But the patient with alcoholic brain damage cannot exercise the will power to quit drinking. He has no insight, and so must be protected from himself or completely restrained from the use of alcohol until reversal of these symptoms from brain damage occurs. Without such preventive procedures, new alcoholics will continue to develop faster than the old ones can be clinically arrested or die off.

Brain damage ushers in a permanent loss of control over alcohol. Such individuals always revert to the uncontrolled pattern whenever they try to drink. At least 50 per cent have associated serious metabolic diseases, especially of the liver, or progressive brain damage, and atrophy of the frontal lobes of the brain, which govern the higher intellectual centers. If the individual goes on untreated at this stage, he becomes an alcoholic derelict, with progressive liver disease or psychotic deterioration, and ends up on skid row, a mental hospital, or in early death.

In the programming of the many symposia on alcoholism, the most neglected field is the relation of alcoholic intoxication, chronic abuse, and true addiction to brain diseases. For example, the symposium held under the auspices of the National Council on Alcoholism, published by the New York Academy of Medicine in 1973, was on alcoholism and the central nervous system, which seemed pointed in the right direction, yet even in this comprehensive group of studies, covering anatomic, physiologic, biochemical and neurologic sequelae of nervous system involvement, the practical application of this basic science knowledge to treatment of alcoholism was ignored. No paper on this important aspects was given.

Classification of Alcoholic Brain Disorders

(1) Acute brain syndrome, withdrawal syndrome. Delirium tremens or acute hallucinosis.

(2) Intermediate stage of alcoholic brain disease. Chronic mental deterioration.

(3) Simple progressive dementia, paranoidal type.

(4) Advanced Korsakoff's/Wernicke's syndrome.

One cannot separate neurologic and psychiatric disorders caused by alcoholism. One of the great oversights in the voluminous literature on alcoholism is the neglect of neurologic involvement. This is partly because many sociologists and psychologists write about alcoholism without knowledge of the importance of neurology. Also, many psychodynamically oriented psychiatrists are not sufficiently trained in organic aspects of brain disorders and thus seem incapable of detecting signs of organicity in patients' behavior, looking only for psychological explanations. A vast number of addictive alcoholics with personality disorders or even psychoses are never detected. They are everywhere, in jails, on skid rows, covered up by families in their homes, or hopeless tramps or transients moving from place to place. A small number are in halfway shelters, cared for by agencies such as the Salvation Army, religious centers or Alcoholics Anonymous.

These unfortunates show the typical signs after a few days of drinking following a short period of abstinence, or after prolonged drinking and several days of abstinence. The symptoms are similar to barbital intoxication and sudden withdrawal. The picture has been reproduced in animals following abrupt withdrawal after two months of administration of ethanol—showing true physiologic addictive phenomena. Formerly these disorders were often fatal (about 15 to 20 per cent). In recent years, with better treatment, the fatality is practically nil unless other serious complications are present. I know of no proved preventive treatment. Cases of latent grand mal or psychomotor epilepsy may show acute symptoms from alcohol. Convulsive disorders of epileptic type may be hard to differentiate from alcohol-induced convulsions. If they are followed by delirium, they are usually alcohol-induced.

Alcoholics with sleep disorders may be on the verge of delirium or convulsions. Bakeland and Lundwall [32] confirm this in studies on sleep disturbances in alcoholics. Patients with blackouts who slept poorly indicated early brain damage. Delirium tremens patients had poorer sleep, suggestive of physical dependency, while those without withdrawal symptoms were anxiety-induced. EEG examinations would probably show abnormalities of a convulsive pattern in physically dependent cases.

Chronic Brain Syndrome

The clinical symptoms of the intermediate stage of alcoholic brain disease are manifest in this condition.

The personality changes in persons with intermediate stage brain damage include rationalization of drinking, pathologic lying, infantile behavior, poor judgment, hostility, emotional liability and lack of insight. The drinking pattern is addictive, dependent or compulsive, usually with daytime and solitary drinking. Among the physiologic reactions are included blackouts, withdrawal reactions and severe hangovers. There are delirious or convulsive episodes in about 50 per cent of cases, and systemic complications such as fatty liver, cirrhosis, and polyneuritis. The main findings of the psychological tests are perceptual (visual), organizational defect, intellectual and personality deterioration and impaired power of abstraction. As already described in a previous chapter, electroencephalographic, tomographic and pneumoencephalographic studies can be carried out to reveal evidence of cerebral atrophy.

Progressive chronic mental deterioration: Although some patients have chronic mental deterioration without acute convulsive episodes, delirium or hallucinations, but their disease is undoubtedly from progressive cerebral atrophy. These individuals lose their ethical and moral values, become insensitive to the feelings of others, and are careless in personal dress and hygiene and social customs. Their behavior is crude. They are inconsiderate, often vulgar and may become abusive and obscene in language. They show gross impairment in intellectual functioning, with defects in memory, judgment and insight. Others who are familiar with their conduct will report progressive personality changes, instability, quarrelsomeness and belligerency; ultimately they become completely incapacitated for useful work. Some, because they resemble cases of paretic dementia, have in the past been classified as alcoholic pseudoparesis. If a pneumogram is obtained, they will show advanced stages of cerebral atrophy. While there may be slight improvement with nutritional and vitamin treatment, the condition is irreversible and hospital confinement may become necessary. They are now making up over 20 per cent of state hospital patients in California, for example, and in increasing numbers are coming in as custodial cases in the Veterans Administration Hospitals.

The Withdrawal Syndrome

Acute alcoholic hallucinosis or delirium tremens: The most important factor in the genesis of delirium tremens and other withdrawal disorders is that it follows a period of chronic intoxication, tremulousness, nausea, retching, motor activity, confusion, disordered sensory perception. These symptoms occur after periods of abstinence. They may be suppressed by a drink or two, but only to recur, with gross tremor and agitation, reaching a peak in 24 hours, with or without convulsions, followed by hallucinations.

Advanced Brain Disease (Wernicke/Korsakoff's Syndrome)

After repeated attacks of delirium, usually associated with malnutrition and vitamin deficiency, persistent spotty memory defects occur with confabulation and emotional lability, from depression to euphoria. These are symptoms of frontal lobe damage or Korsakoff's syndrome. In others, simple progressive dementia may occur, without signs of delirium, but paranoidal persecutory ideation and easy reaction to violence without insight, superficially resembling schizophrenia but with gross sensorial defects, are present. These cases are also allied to pathologic intoxication with convulsive episodes induced by alcohol.

The Korsakoff-Wernicke syndromes are essentially the same, and have been shown to be hemorrhagic encephalopathies from vitamin deficiency. They also have been described in avitaminotic states without alcohol. Usually, associated neurologic aculomotor palsies, nystagmus and peripheral polyneuropathies are present. Recent memory loss is most striking, with the patient unable to recall events occurring a few minutes before, with fanciful tales (confabulation) to fill in the memory gaps. This stage usually means irreversible brain damage has occurred. General physical and neurologic improvement may occur with proper nutrition and vitamin therapy, but constant supervision and protection from alcoholic exposure is required to prevent relapse or further intellectual detioration.

CHAPTER SEVEN

Developing Constructive Relationships between Psychiatry, General Medicine and Alcoholics Anonymous

Many physicians do not accept alcoholic patients and feel no medical responsibility for them. They ignore or cooperate very little with Alcoholics Anonymous, which for 40 years has had success in treating alcoholics. Likewise, members of Alcoholics Anonymous often strongly resist working with doctors and with patients under medical treatment; they criticize medical therapies and discredit emotional factors as a cause of alcoholism. The result is gross and continuing neglect of the problem. These differing attitudes of physicians and lay workers weaken or hamper efforts at treatment and rehabilitation of alcoholics and research. There is a scarcity of doctors and hospitals that regularly treat alcoholic patients.

To gain a better understanding of these problems a symposium was held at the American Psychiatric Association meeting, Los Angeles, on May 5, 1964,* covering various aspects of the need for cooperation between Alcoholics Anonymous and psychiatric facilities for treatment of alcoholism. The following opinions were condensed from tape recordings of the discussions.

The Moderator was A. E. Bennett, Director of the A. E. Bennett Neuropsychiatric Research Foundation, who gave the reasons for the symposium:

For the past fifteen years a major interest of my Foundation has been research in alcoholism, for which an award was received from the American Medical Association for research on Alcoholic Brain Disease. Psychiatrists and medical practitioners tend not to accept or treat alcoholics. The medical

* The opinions of the participants expressed in 1964 are still valid. The principal changes since then are: much greater acceptance that alcoholism is a treatable disease, more general hospitals accept alcoholic patients, including Veterans Administration hospitals, providing in and out patient facilities. A national institute on alcoholism and alcoholic abuse was established in 1970, and in 1974 congressional legislation provided 350 million dollars for pioneering work in treatment. The National Council on Alcoholism and the American Association on Alcoholism (800 physician members) merged in 1974. Health insurance programs are increasingly giving minimal coverage for treatment. The biggest problem is still to get more physicians to understand and adequately treat the disease. Uniform laws have been adopted by two-fifths of the states, providing in part that public drunks be sent to treatment facilities rather than to jail. (CAMA Newsletter, March 3, 1975, p. 4.)

profession and Alcoholics Anonymous fail to understand each other's goals and methods and how constructive relationships can be developed between them. The panel participants from psychiatry, general medicine and Alcoholics Anonymous explored various facets of the problem, suggesting methods of cooperation and other improvements.

Mrs. Marty Mann, the Founder and Executive Director of the National Council on Alcoholism, at this meeting was made an Honorary Fellow of the American Psychiatric Association. She discussed how AA works and how psychiatric and general medical practitioners fail to understand it. She suggested an educative program to bring the two groups closer together in a cooperative treatment program that could reach thousands of patients.

Keith Ditman, Director of Alcoholism Research at the University of California at Los Angeles, discussed the failure of psychiatrists to comprehensively treat the alcoholic and to use AA help; conversely, he also indicated how AA can better understand psychiatry's role. Paul O'Halloran, of the Shadel Institute in Seattle, represented a private hospital that has pioneered outstanding techniques in the successful treatment of thousands of alcoholics. He discussed how to achieve better coordination in treatment between AA and private hospitals. Jackson Smith, a former member of the American Medical Association Council on Alcoholism and of a Committee of State Hospital Management of Alcoholism, explained the role of the A.M.A. in educating the medical profession in public health aspects of alcoholism, and described hospital programs that better utilize AA in treatment.

Karl E. Voldeng represented the successful nonpsychiatric practitioners' treatment of the alcoholic. A surgeon active in Kansas State Programs for many years, now in private practice in Phoenix, he has a wide and successful experience in the treatment of alcoholics and is author of a practical book, "Recovery from Alcoholism" (H. Regnery Co., Chicago, 1962).

The Moderator's opening remarks noted: I have worked with AA since its beginning, with many former patients establishing chapters, and have relied heavily upon them in the joint management of seriously ill alcoholic patients. At the same time, I have been conscious of the fact that most physicians do not like to treat alcoholic patients and believe there is little that can be done for them. Many psychiatrists refuse to accept them. These concerns about medicine's neglect of the problem and awareness of what the doctors and AA together can do in the total rehabilitation of the alcoholic came into direct focus while I was lecturing in Honolulu. After addressing AA members, questions arose on how general physicians and psychiatrists could be oriented to accept AA philosophy. It appeared that the AA in Hawaii was receiving practically no medical help. I became more aware of the fact that doctors are not oriented toward alcoholism as a treatable illness.

They are not trained to deal with it as a disease and as a rule do not regard themselves as having any responsibility to people addicted to alcohol. These observations led me to the idea that something should be done to establish a better understanding of AA within the medical profession. The best way to start seemed to obtain authoritative sponsorship of an educational forum. This resulted in enlisting the aid of a panel of experts to gather before the American Psychiatric Associations for a Round Table Meeting. The picture of medical and/or psychiatric treatment of the alcoholic in most localities is very bleak. This most serious public health problem receives very little attention in practice by our profession, in spite of the AMA resolution of 1956 that alcoholism is a disease and therefore a medical responsibility.

A special research group set up by the National Council on Alcoholism to study conditions in New York City reported as follows: The medical and other professions are grossly unaware of or indifferent to the problems and show little interest in treating or understanding the alcoholic; the view of alcoholism as a disease is far from being accepted. Only four hospitals in New York accept alcoholics as patients. Of the 258,000 alcoholics only 52,000 get any kind of help at all.*

17% of general practitioners, 21% of internists and 31% of psychiatrists refuse to treat alcoholism. This situation is probably similar in most states and cities. Alcoholics Anonymous has proved more continuously successful than doctors in treating the alcoholic. In 25 years it grew to about 300,000 (by 1975 to 800,000) members. Yet they are reaching less than 10% of the number they should be serving. It is estimated that the disease is increasing at the rate of 200,000 new alcoholics each year. AA would grow much faster if all doctors who treat alcoholics would cooperate with local AA chapters. I believe that if we can adequately present the facts to the medical profession we can break down the present pessimistic attitude and get large numbers of doctors to accept responsibility in the problem of treating alcoholics.

Why does psychiatry so often fail with alcoholics? The following statement from an alcoholic in sustained sobriety with AA reflects a common complaint about the failure of psychiatric treatment.

"I went to a psychiatrist for more than four years, intermittently, seeking help for my drinking problem. During the course of treatment I continued to drink, even while experiencing social, economic and moral difficulties as a result of drinking." Another common complaint was that these patients hoped their psychiatrist would find and eliminate the roots of their problem and thus the desire to drink, that once the cause of the disorder were uncovered, the problem of alcoholism would be automatically solved.

Alcoholics generally seem to believe that psychiatric treatment is ineffective.

---

* Treatment facilities have improved since these figures of 1964. See footnote on opening page of this chapter.

Psychiatrists are often made fun of, or arouse fears within the patient that they will be treated as insane or that commitment will be recommended. Are patients justified in this attitude about psychiatry? Other questions immediately arise. Why do so many psychiatrists refuse to treat alcoholics? Do they lack training to adequately treat the alcoholic? Are we naive or gullible? Does the psychiatrist fail to understand the problem? Are his techniques faulty? Would better understanding of AA and closer working relationships help in the rehabilitation? Does the psychiatrist fail to utilize other aids properly, relying too much on psychotherapy? These and other questions we hoped to get answers to in our discussion period.

Next why does the general practitioner usually fail to relieve alcoholism? AA state that their loss of confidence in the average doctor's treatment is because the great bulk of treatment consists of shots or pills directed towards symptoms. They feel that doctors don't seem motivated to attempt to cope with the problem of alcoholism. The doctor doesn't seem interested in or understand AA and is critical of the organization. The alcoholic recognizes that he arouses feelings of anger, futility or disgust on the part of the doctor, which prevents rapport, and the doctor can't handle these situations and attitudes. In AA there is the attitude of sympathetic hopefulness. The alcoholic feels understood, and communication is established. He learns complete surrender to AA philosophy as a way of life to maintain sobriety. Are these criticisms of the average medical practitioner justified? Do many doctors fail to diagnose and properly treat alcoholics, lack the training properly to understanding alcoholism as a disease? Do doctors really admit the alcoholic is sick? If the doctor considers his patient an outcast, he can't have sincere understanding and be helpful. If this is indeed the case, how can we change these attitudes and enlist the aid of general practitioners to become more conscious of alcoholism and look for alcoholic addiction as the cause of many of their patients' problems. With proper knowledge they may reach the compulsive drinker with the awareness that for him, only one drink stands between health and sickness.

Next, where does AA fail to understand medicine's contribution to treatment. It has been claimed that AA is not as effective as formerly, that there is a widening gap between AA and scientists. Some criticize AA's attitude about alcoholics who can't adopt AA and state that AA is hostile to criticism, that AA thinking dominates public education, that the organization takes authoritative stands on medical therapy and is critical of drugs, for example, tranquilizers. Many members, indeed, are critical of disulfiram (Antabuse) to control drinking, and many refuse to accept that emotional illness plays any part in alcoholism. These attitudes hinder recovery and scientific research. AA dogma is said to be too rigid and fanatical and that the organization is too satisfied with the arrested recovery and continued dependency on AA, instead of realizing that many other programs help. It has also been stated that AA is a way to obtain sobriety, but that this is not the whole answer and that other treatments succeed where AA fails and vice versa. With these generalizations of the problem, many controversial points are raised. The panel participants enlarged on these and many other points and attempted to clarify misunderstanding and offer suggestions for solutions.

Dr. Keith S. Ditman discussed psychiatrists' failure in the comprehensive treatment of the alcoholic and lack of utilization of AA; criticisms of AA; and suggestions of how the psychiatrist might be persuaded to treat alcoholism.

The concept of alcoholism certainly is changing from a moral to a medical one, and there are numerous factors contributing to this change. Many of them have to do with advances in the field of medicine itself. With developments in psychotherapy, sociology and psychopharmacology, the role of the physician has radically changed, and his services have become crucial in conditions previously not considered within his province. There is an explosive amount of research in the field of mental health, including alcoholism. Many important findings are being made, but not immediately put into practice because of limitations of time and techniques for postgraduate education. New findings to be integrated into the practice of medicine often have to be introduced at the start of the physician's training, which is a long and slow process. Thus, it may take a decade or more for an important discovery to be commonly used in practice. Let me give an example.

Over ten years ago the phenothiazine tranquilizer, chlorpromazine, was found to have antipsychotic properties. Yet today many physicians do not believe in its use in the treatment of acute schizophrenia despite evidence to the contrary. For example, the recent NIMH hospital study showed it effective in about 95% of acute schizophrenics.

Its inclusion into the practice of the physicians' treatment for alcoholism is similarly a slow process. Although psychiatry has moved slowly in this field, I don't view it as a failure. Alcoholism as a subspecialty in psychiatry is still viable and thriving, and I expect acceleration of its growth in the very near future. There are many things that can be done to hasten this process. I'm not so sure that energizing the psychiatrists is what I would put first on the list. Perhaps most important is incorporation of alcoholism into the medical school curriculum, and clinical experience in the treatment of the alcoholic. It is also important to include these in residency training programs in psychiatry and internal medicine, as it is from these groups that will come those who will do much of the teaching and research on alcoholism in the future. To build a large pool of alcoholism specialists trained in all the techniques that can be used with alcoholics takes considerable time, but is badly needed.

The second thing that could be provided is postgraduate courses for physicians and paramedical personnel in the techniques of treating and managing the alcoholic. Since alcoholism is a condition requiring treatment, the physician should be the primary individual responsible for the treatment. After all, the physician is the one licensed to practice medicine, and if alcoholism is a disease, for non-physicians to assume responsibility for treatment of the alcoholic would perhaps be practicing medicine without a license. Although some alcoholics will respond to acceptance or simple counsel, obviously most of them do not. Many of the other useful methods of treatment of alcoholics can be prescribed or properly supervised only by the physician. Alcoholism is a serious problem and I see no reason why it should be given second rate or only partial treatment. Although there is yet much to be learned about the condition, we do know that even many difficult cases will respond to a combination of treatments. These treatments include various psychotherapies, medicines, drugs such as Antabuse, the psychopharmacologic agents, participation in the Alcoholics Anonymous program and the use of such techniques as that of treatment probation by the employer and the court. Currently in California, the use of summary probation by the court to treatment is gaining considerable recognition by many judges and psychiatrists as a valuable technique. Our own investigations in this area indicate that court referred patients are good risks to stay sober. As new discoveries are made in the field of medicine and psychiatry, these too can be incorporated into the treatment of the alcoholic by the physician.

The third thing is to increase the interest of the physician and psychiatrist in treating the alcoholic. One is to fully integrate the alcoholic patient in medical and psychiatric settings. This is being done at the Neuropsychiatric Institute at UCLA and the alcoholic patient is as welcome as a neurotic, psychotic or a character disorder. This has taken place over the past two years. Just as hospitals have units for contagious diseases and psychiatric patients, the psychiatric unit needs to be designed in such a way that it fulfills the needs of the suicidal patient, the acute psychotic, the alcoholic and many other types of patients. Many alcoholic patients say that during their alcoholic withdrawal it is disturbing to be put in with schizophrenics, and they have voiced what they thought of the doctor for doing this. Because of the way hospitals are structured, however, it has not been possible to put them elsewhere. Hospitals should be designed for the patients and not for the people who design them. They should be run for the patients and not for the people who run them. Unfortunately, this is not always the case.

The integration of the treatment of the alcoholic into medical and psychiatric training of the physician and the integration of treatment of the alcoholic into medical and psychiatric hospitals is necessary for a competent, complete treatment program of all types of alcoholic problems. Besides competency of treatment there are reasons for integrating the alcoholic into the physician-hospital treatment program. One of them is the changing nature of programs for medical care and disability payments. Private insurance carriers, a growing segment of the medical care program, are just beginning to include psychiatric conditions for patient care. There is no reason why alcoholism should not be included in such coverage.

The real question in the field of alcoholism is whether it will complete the process of becoming a professional problem and be accepted as such. There are many paramedical and lay approaches for the treatment of the alcoholic that have been invaluable in the past. Most outstanding has been the fellowship of Alcoholics Anonymous. This organization has helped many alcoholics but by no means all. Like most treatments, it is only one of many and frequently can be used best when combined with others. Just as there has been an anti-professional lethargy concerning the alcoholic, there has been an anti-professional attitude on the part of some AA members as well.

Recently there have been several articles suggesting that this anti-professionalism on the part of Alcoholics Anonymous is increasing. For example, a pamphlet published by Alcoholics Anonymous entitled "Tranquilizers, Sedatives and the Alcoholic" presented the argument that the alcoholic should never take any of these drugs, even when prescribed by a physician. They state this recommendation is presented as a "suggestion" gained from summing up many personal experiences and meaningful case histories and not as a "dogmatic rule," even though "the testimony may be clear and impressive." Most of this attitude toward drugs was formed in the early days of the fellowship, before the advent of the phenothiazine tranquilizers, for example, and is now applied without change, as far as I can tell, to all the newer drugs. It is stated in this pamphlet that there is "considerable support in current medical literature" for the conclusion that all of these drugs are harmful to the alcoholic. References are not cited. In the beginning of the pamphlet there are statements to the effect that (1) pills never help with problems and emotional tension; (2) new tranquilizing drugs and alcoholics are incompatible; (3) any substance that affects the nervous system in the long run will be addictable; and (4) the alcoholic should avoid the long continued use of any drug since he will get into trouble. Although it is mentioned that staying free of any chemical support is the broader goal, they fail to point out that not all alcoholics are the same and that some suffer from mental conditions for which short or long continued use of some of the newer drugs is effective. Certainly one would not expect a diabetic to do without insulin, and the effectiveness of the phenothiazine tranquilizers for some major mental illnesses is well documented. One could hardly expect alcoholics who are schizophrenic to do without a drug that can help them. Furthermore, the discomforts and deaths from the alcoholic withdrawal syndrome have been greatly reduced by the tranquilizers, sedatives and anticonvulsants. This pamphlet and other AA literature indicates that AA wants the alcoholic to stay away from drugs, which are like alcohol for him in their addictive properties. The point that the alcoholic is an addiction-prone person is well known. It is recognized in medicine and AA that barbiturates are addictive, and have no place in the long-term treatment of the alcoholic. The single exception is phenobarbital for persons suffering from epilepsy. Alcoholics often suffer from chronic emotional and mental problems, in addition to their problem of drinking. The pamphlet says nothing about this, nor the need for drug treatment of alcoholics with schizophrenia and severe depression which, if untreated, could end in severe phobias, periodic panic attacks, or suicide.

All of these conditions can often be treated successfully with drugs. Not only does the pamphlet omit mention of them and the possibility of their drug treatment, it implies that anyone taking drugs is cheating and guilty of hypocrisy for not finding his entire answer in AA.

At the UCLA Alcoholism Research Clinic we have treated several thousands of alcoholics with drugs; rarely do the patients misuse them and not one case of addiction to these drugs has appeared. AA's statement about "Our many friends in the field of medicine not all of whom may today be fully in accord with the tone of this pamphlet" is quite right, as much of it is anti-physician and certainly all of it is anti-drug.

The insistence on the AA program alone, the requirement for a conscious contact with a higher power for the alcoholic to be able to solve his problems, and the avoidance of all drugs undoubtedly works for some, perhaps many, but not all alcoholics. Such a point of view of a single approach can only be the result of a misconception of the emotional and mental problems some alcoholics have, as well as a confusion regarding drugs. For example, in the pamphlet a popular, not a scientific, use of the term "tranquilizers" is used. Under "tranquilizers" are lumped sedatives known to be addicting, as well as phenothiazine, which is not addicting. This implication that tranquilizers are addicting then carries through the rest of the pamphlet. The drugs that are specifically named in six case histories are known to be addicting, and from the definition given to tranquilizers a lay reader could easily conclude that all these drugs are addicting, too. However, in the case histories, no phenothiazine tranquilizer, no anticonvulsant or antidepressant drug is specifically mentioned.

Physicians treating alcoholics are increasingly finding it of value to refer them to AA as part of the treatment program. Psychiatrists are also agreeing more that AA is of value for the alcoholic and frequently refer them. Such patients are often placed in a conflict situation when additional treatment, including drugs and psychotherapy, are used by the physician. The physician must be prepared to help the patient resolve this conflict and understand the nature and reasons for his medication. It would also be of help if AA incorporated in their literature material more accurately informing the alcoholic with regards to drugs and their proper use in treatment. In a previous pamphlet, no longer issued by the AA organization, they express a less nihilistic attitude toward physicians and drugs. They said "It is one thing to prescribe AA for the uncomplicated alcoholic who is ready to try any port in a storm. It's quite another to assume an all-knowing wisdom where the far more complex factors of drugs are present. The latter is a job for competent medical practitioners exclusively." "The AA who attains his sense of values will recognize that his only gift is the priceless one of his experience in arresting his drinking problem. His sobriety newly acquired or carefully nurtured over a period of years no more entitles him to prescribe for the pill user than it would qualify him to operate for cancer."

In conclusion let me say that it should be recognized that alcoholism is a ubiquitous difficult problem, and no person or group has the entire answer. Physicians do find AA fellowship helpful for some of their patients, and many members of AA have benefited from medical care for their emotional problems. The insistence on one approach and exclusion of others can only hurt many alcoholics and hinder the progress of treatment. Needed are greater efforts and more cooperation from the medical profession, research and training centers, and Alcoholics Anonymous in the treatment and understanding of alcoholism.

Discussion

Dr. Jackson Smith:* The AMA has attempted in the past, and I presume will continue to try in the future, to stimulate interest in alcoholism in State and County medical groups. To accomplish this, the AMA has repeatedly sponsored symposia on the subject. They have a scientific exhibit on alcoholism, which is sent over the country throughout the year, attempting to encourage the local doctor to treat these people as a part of his medical responsibility. In 1956 there was a resolution passed by the House of Delegates, which said that these patients should be admitted to general hospitals without exclusion on the basis of diagnosis. The major intent of this resolution was to increase the acceptance of alcoholics as a medical responsibility and to officially clarify the AMA's opposition to their exclusion from general hospitals.

It was hoped this effort would offer a more reliable index of the admission of alcoholics to general hospitals and increase the insurance coverage available to such patients.

The AMA also works with the Council of Medical Education to encourage the inclusion of courses on alcoholism in the medical school curriculums. The

* Jackson Smith, Professor of Psychiatry, Loyola University, Stritch School of Medicine, Chicago, Ill.

subject is usually discussed in three departments: medicine, public health and psychiatry. Deciding what should be taught about alcoholism is not a question dulled by accord. Everyone agrees the alcoholic should be treated; but not everyone is overly clear about the content of courses for medical students. One reason for discord may arise from the fact that this is undoubtedly the most frequently and variously cured group of people in the world. This applies both during recovery from a drinking bout and periods of sobriety.

The patient who is repeatedly admitted to State Hospitals, is one who is arrested, committed, briefly sobered and repeats the cycle. He is usually a homeless man without family, material possessions or responsibility, and sobriety is a function of his environment. It doesn't arise from within himself. In other words, if alcohol is available, he will drink; if it isn't, he adapts rather well to his surroundings. The cycle of arrest and commitment, physical recovery and discharge back to Skid Row is hardly the answer. This isn't very popular to suggest at the moment, but it would seem that each time he's committed, he should be kept for a longer period of time. There are people who are unable to function in a community and until methods of treatment improve, there is little else for them but to restrict their environments.

For those alcoholics who are neither psychotic nor suffering from organic brain damage, I feel very strongly than an open ward in a state hospital with work assignments as well as group therapy is quite beneficial.

Dr. Karl E. Voldeng:* Where I practice there has been a considerable increase in medical interest toward the alcoholic patient in the past few years. The doctors are interested and there is a definite trend toward the treatment of those in trouble. I will briefly outline my method of handling the alcoholic who comes into my office. Realize that this outline is one followed by internists and G.P's, or, in other words, the non-psychiatrists in this community who try to help the alcoholic.

My first concern is to show the patient that I am sincerely anxious to help in any medical way possible, whatever the illness may be. I try to demonstrate sincerity and friendliness. I try to reflect a definite sympathy. I emphasize the fact that I am a doctor.

I suggest to the patient that I should know more about him and be able to observe and study him more thoroughly before launching into a schedule of therapy.

I try to get these patients into the hospital, because I am convinced that a week or two will afford opportunities for a successful rehabilitation that cannot be obtained on an outpatient basis. The hospital period offers an opportunity

* Karl E. Voldeng, private practice in general medicine and surgery, especially active in alcoholism treatment in Phoenix, Ariz.

for a complete medical investigation. It also places the patient in an atmosphere most conductive to the process of "drying out." It gives me an opportunity to get a clear picture of the patient and I have visits with the wife or members of the family in an effort to more completely evaluate the circumstances. I try to investigate every angle from both the physical and functional standpoints.

Finally comes the time when the diagnosis is discussed with the patient. This includes every facet of his medical profile, including the functional elements and the behavior pattern involving use of alcohol.

As the patient reaches his first stage of sobriety, I discuss with him help available in Alcoholics Anonymous. I inform the patient that a member of AA will visit him in the hospital, and the AA member chosen for this assignment is selected on the basis of qualifications and status to fit that of the patient. I also discuss with the patient my medical opinion as to the importance of a religious fellowship. This discussion is immediately followed by a visitation from a clergyman suitable for this specialized form of ministry.

Both the members of AA and the ministry continue their close association with the patient. The patient often is taken out to an AA meeting during the last few days of his hospital stay. These associations are carefully continued as the patient is dismissed from the hospital.

As the physician, I explain in detail the nature of alcoholism, the disease pattern, and the necessity for sobriety. I stress the fact that in his particular case alcohol must be completely avoided. I explain this fact in no uncertain terms, with the same emphasis that I would chart the do's and don't's for a diabetic, a peptic ulcer patient, or one with a recent coronary occlusion.

From a psychological standpoint I stress the fact that rather than something being taken away from his life, he is on the threshold of having may new things added to his life, which will bring happiness and health unknown to him in recent years. The program of rehabilitation is then outlined to encompass precisely this philosophy.

After dismissal from the hospital the patient is closely followed by his doctor, AA contacts, and the Church. He is given every possible support and encouragement.

There is a small hospital in Phoenix devoted entirely to the treatment of alcoholism. Medical men have the privilege of utilizing this facility of referring an alcoholic patient to the care of their staff. AA also maintains rehabilitation homes for both men and women.

I would say that approximately 10 per cent of the patients that I see eventually disclose psychotic manifestations, which are cause for referral to a psychiatrist and a transfer to that specialized field of therapy. Even with such a transfer I usually try to keep in touch with the patient, chiefly on the basis of personal interest. The psychiatrist seems happy to have a general medical man keeping an eye on possible organic complications. Another 10 per cent are sent for psychiatric evaluation and the psychiatrist's suggestions are used in continuing therapy.

*Dr. Paul O'Hollaren** (representing a private hospital which treats alcoholism exclusively): It is a real pleasure to hear this gradual amalgamation of the different disciplines taking place. A lot of our patients tried AA and failed. They would go to AA afterwards and needle friends who had failed on AA. This generated hostility. I think Marty Mann is correct when she says that in those days the doctors just would not accept the alcoholic patient, even under any consideration with this attitude, and we could well expect the AA to move in.

The one common denominator we've all missed is the failure to unify our research efforts. Anonymity in AA, I think, for research purposes has become passé. In the first place, alcoholism is no longer a disease you have to hide, as if you had a "social disease."

Getting different disciplines to recognize needs for hospitalization and complete care, when the patient has been drinking two fifths a day for 60 to 90 days, is a big problem. Just trying to talk him out of drinking and telling him to come in and have a shot of vitamin B three times a week is futile and dangerous. Rather, we have to get him into a hospital facility at this early stage of treatment, have him dried out, before trying to talk to him. Then you can start the psychiatric approach, and the patient is then the best subject for AA, too. Omission of these preliminary measures accounts for a lot of AA failures. Most of our patients have been to AA; when asked why they don't or couldn't carry on—"I was just too sick . . . I couldn't sit there and listen . . .".

I think we should unite different disciplines in a unified approach to research. If everybody is working for one goal the chances of success are enhanced. With the help of the American Psychiatric Association and others in the field of alcoholism willing to participate, we whip this disease.

Questions From the Audience

Question for Dr. Smith: Why do you think a work detail is helpful for hospitalized alcoholics? Many of these tasks are demeaning.

Answer: I don't think they are demeaning. Many alcoholics get very restless sitting around the hospital ward, waiting for time to pass. I am aware that in the past they almost ran some state hospitals and became so essential that the

* Paul O'Hollaren, Medical Director, Shadel Hospital for Alcoholism, Seattle, Wash.

staff was reluctant to discharge them. I don't think these tasks are demeaning any more than being a psychiatrist may be demeaning; for that matter, psychiatrists might profit from a few work assignments, too. Alcoholics become restless sitting around, and are gratified by what they are given to do and take pride in it.

Question for Dr. Smith: Would a nationwide education of the public health aspects of alcoholism be helpful, somewhat like that which is going on now for tobacco in relation to cancer?

Answer: Since 1937 the alcoholics have gone from being drunks, to AA members, to being a medical problem. I think one of medicine's greatest contributions to this problem has been mentioned, that it dignifies the illness. If you are sick it is all right to admit that you are sick. Now as to how education is to be carried on—this is out of my area, but this is the way I feel. I think much has been done. As far as I know, AA members are the only people who have gotten together to help themselves, in a well organized way, because they have a particular illness. I am much encouraged by AA's efforts to educate. I think they work very well in most locales with the Council on Alcoholism. These people help by giving information and a number to call which will contact AA and/or hospitals that will take alcoholic patients.

Question for Dr. O'Hollaren: What do you do to get the resistant alcoholic into treatment?

Answer: This is one of the biggest problems facing all of us. Informants say, "He knows he has a problem," but the patient doesn't want to do anything about it. Dr. Lemere and I did a study in which we found that 65 per cent of the patients were under duress. They were there because they had the "or else" treatment by the wife, the boss, or minister. This duress we thought for a long time was bad. There is a common saying among alcoholics that you can't help an alcoholic who doesn't want to be helped. I don't agree with that. We have had a really good success ratio in the duress group. We should face this thing from a legal standpoint. We have to have legislation in this disease sooner or later. We took 285 prisoners from the courts out of the State Prison of Idaho over a ten year period. We had an 81 per cent success ratio in those that came out of the court—61 per cent in total abstinence, with no violation; the FBI checked those who came out of prison. Now this is duress at its best. These persons could see that sobriety meant a lot to them. So I think we are going to have to come around to some type of duress. Why should an alcoholic, who won't face his problem, be allowed to get on freeways? We do it by encouraging the wife or others close to him to put the pressure on. The wife always says, "I'll leave." And then the fellow drinks up the house. I tell her, if you are really fed up with failing to make this decision, get a restraining order and move him out. "I love you dearly, darling—BUT—with one hand—BUT you either take treatments and straighten out—or else!" It's amazing how often that works.

Question for Marty Mann:* At what stage in the alcoholic's recovery should the patient be referred to AA by the psychiatrist?

Answer: Frankly I don't think you can give just one answer to that. I think this varies with patients and I think the psychiatrist is usually the best judge. If the psychiatrist is knowledgable about AA and has some techniques of doing this kind of referral, I think he will know best at what point this should be done. I just don't see how that could be answered in general, for all alcoholics.

Question: Would it depend pretty much on the patient's attitude about AA?

Answer: I think a good deal. I was very interested in hearing Dr. Ruth Fox, a psychiatrist who knows a good deal about the treatment of alcoholics, state that in a number of cases the question of getting the patient to go to AA had been rather a long-term proposition. It often takes considerable time and effort and the therapist has a responsibility to motivate the patient to do this. She accepts that responsibility and makes definite efforts to get the alcoholic first to accept any kind of treatment and, when the time came, to accept AA as well.

Question for Marty Mann: If alcoholics are not joiners would this explain why AA had success with less than 10 per cent of the alcoholics?

Answer: I think there is an indirect inference there. The figure that we use for the number of alcoholics is around 5,000,000 at least. Even the most conservative figure is between 4 and 5 million. You earlier heard the figure mentioned for members of AA as 300,000. Now that is quite a lot less than 10 per cent of 5 million. But I don't think you can say that AA has not had success with that other 90 per cent and more because they have never been to AA. It hasn't had success because there has been no contact. I don't believe that if a person has never been to a psychiatrist you can say that psychiatry had failed with that person. I believe that this matter of alcoholics not being joiners certainly has contributed to keeping lots of people from trying AA in the first place or going near it. One of the points that I wanted to make earlier and I didn't get to it was that in many cases we have to build bridges to the alcoholic. The alcoholic is not, as a general rule, running down the street screaming for help all the time. I don't go along with the fact that we have to wait until he falls from a tree like a ripe plum because a ripe plum usually squashes on the ground and is no good for eating or anything . . . if you wait till it falls. I

---

* Marty Mann, founder and Executive Director of the National Council on Alcoholism. Author of the widely read "New Primer on Alcoholism": Holt, Rinehart and Winston, New York, 1958.

believe that we must find many ways of getting alcoholics to treatment before they think they are ready for it. There are ways and I don't think we have to depend entirely on legal methods, although I think these may be useful in many cases. There are other methods with which people can be brought into treatment. Of the many thousands of AA members that I know, I can count on my fingers the ones I know that went willingly. AA is responsible for their help, but they can't help anybody until he wants help. And yet very few go willingly. I think almost any alcoholic goes to whatever treatment he goes to under duress. It's not always the same kind of duress. You've heard quite a number of types mentioned here. There is another type of duress that hasn't been mentioned. A lot of alcoholics have sought help because of purely social duress. The person who discovers that he is being ostrasized socially, that there are homes his family can no longer go to, that he is not invited to parties anymore and that people don't want him around. This has frequently been the source of motivation to do something. There are many kinds of duress and we don't have to always look to the law. That sounds a little bit like the old Americanism that "There's got to be a law." I think there are other things that could be used and duress can and should be used on most alcoholics. On this business as to why 300,000 alcoholics are known to have recovered out of a possible total population of 5 million alcoholics: I haven't changed the opinion that I have been expressing for 20 years, that the biggest deterrent to seeking help is the stigma that still rests on alcoholism. We haven't eliminated it. It would be awfully nice to think we had. People don't gladly pound their chests and say, "I know what I am, I'm an alcoholic," for all to hear, but more people are seeking help despite the stigma. It has lightened considerably in 20 years, but is not gone. This is certainly not a popular subject, not a popular illness, and the label isn't anything anyone willingly seeks to pin on themselves. It still has not the acceptance and respectability of cancer, tuberculosis, or diabetes, or any other simple physical disease. It shares the same stigma as mental illness, and sometimes the stigma is heavier than for mental illness, sometimes not quite so heavy, but in general it is in the same category. As a matter of fact, people don't like to admit it is in their family. And I think this deterrent keeps the large majority of untreated alcoholics from treatment.

Comment by Dr. O'Hollaren: I don't think it is the stigma, per se, that is the major deterrent. I think it is a tremendous decision for the alcoholic to look ahead and try to envision life without alcohol. We sometimes lose sight of the basic position of the patient—of an individual who has become so utterly dependent on alcohol, who started out as a social drinker, but is now faced with a matter of life and death. He is so frightened at the idea of stopping that he protects his supply, and his whole life is centered around drinking. He is actually deeply frightened, overwhelmed with a sense of self-preservation, the strongest instinct, and the decision to come to treatment or to stop drinking seems impossible because he cannot see the possibility of living without alcohol. That I think is the major thing that keeps alcoholics from going for treatment.

Dr. Ditman:* Mr. Chairman, I would like to take this opportunity to agree with both the speakers. Certainly there is a stigma to alcoholism. No one ever sends a get-well card to an alcoholic! Stigma is a stumbling block, but addiction is a problem too. Look at cigarette smoking. There is no stigma to being a smoker; if anything it is the other way around. Yet few are quitting if you take the incidence of cigarette sales. Smoking is an addictive process and like other addictions the process goes on longer than just during acute withdrawal. The chronicity of alcohol addiction is a good reason for using Antabuse. It can be used for an interpretation to the patient. You can say to the patient, "Do you want to stop?" and he will say, "Yes, of course, why do you think I'm here?" But then you say you can stop right now. "I can?" "If you take Antabuse anybody can stop." Then often he says "Well . . .", and it comes out then that he does not really want to stop. That is the crucial thing in treating the alcoholic—to get him to want to stop. The step before that is to get him to see that he does not want to stop, and even before that is to get him to see that he is an alcoholic and needs to stop. Once you get him to the point where he wants to stop you are a long ways along in treatment.

Dr. Jackson: I agree with Dr. Ditman—to suggest Antabuse is a good test of the sincerity of the individual. But many people are actually very fearful of being without alcohol. "You mean I've got to give it up forever?" I always compromise and say "We'll try it for six months and then talk about it, because to say forever is like saying you can't every smoke again—well, I'd say let's talk about it tomorrow." In 1948 when we first got Antabuse I happened to be in training. It looked so simple to give Antabuse and then people wouldn't drink. Patients can get severe reactions, but this is actually a very safe drug because people don't die of these reactions—at least in my experience. I think it is one of our more effective methods of treatment and is a good test of whether the individual can tolerate sobriety. This is kind of rough on some people.

There is a question whether in nursing training we should include modern approaches to the treatment of the alcoholic. I think we should, because nurses are in very close contact with this type of patient. The patient again, ordinarily if he is an alcoholic, will talk to the individual he is most at ease with, which may well be the nurse. She should know what she has to handle. Another question is whether or not a recovered alcoholic should be a counselor in the alcoholic unit. Of course this would be ideal if you had the right individual each

---

* Keith S. Ditman, M.D., Professor of Psychiatry, University of California at Los Angeles, and Director of Alcoholic Research Center.

time. Most state hospitals will allow AA to send someone in to suit their needs. In my own experience AA has always been most cooperative.

Question for Dr. Voldeng: How frequently do you feel the diagnosis of alcoholism is missed by the average physician?

Answer: I think it is missed very frequently. I saw just a few days ago that someone in general hospitals had gone over the patient census on a particular day and they found a tremendous number of alcoholics all over the hospital. Yet there was nothing on the record about it. The intern or the resident or the staff man had said nothing about it. I think the diagnosis is completely missed primarily because the staff doesn't think of it. The doctor would just as soon not think of it and the patient would just as soon not discuss it and so there is no reason to even bring it up, and it is just sort of side-stepped so it just doesn't exist as far as records are concerned.

Dr. Bennett: I would like to add that in our studies in alcoholism devoted particularly to the brain function we found that many medical men and psychiatrists did not recognize chronic organic changes in the brain in alcoholism. It is a very important thing to diagnose early alcoholic brain disease and not just to treat these symptoms as neurotic manifestations. These personality changes are the result of definite frontal lobe disease. And that's part of the diagnostic problem. Until the organic brain syndrome clears up you cannot get motivation and you cannot get any other therapies under way. Sometimes that rehabilitating process takes many weeks or months. And that is our big problem, how to control that alcoholic in sobriety who has brain damage until reversibility occurs, if it will reverse. We have ways of finding that out, we have published our research studies upon this aspect of alcoholism.

Question for Dr. Ditman: Do you think the average citizen knows the difference between the many drugs now in use? Aren't the majority of AA members average citizens? How can AA be educated in such fine points?

Answer: I think and hope that AA members are average citizens. And it is certainly true that most people do not know the difference between various drugs or tranquilizers. But they should know that not all drugs are addicting and when in doubt should be encouraged to consult medical advice. The thing I was talking about is the information put out by the AA organization, i.e., the red pamphlet, and this is done with the help of consultants. What is really necessary is that this information be accurate, understandable and kept up to date. Actually what appears to have developed during the time between those two pamphlets I mentioned is a tendency to become ingrained in an anti-drug attitude. I think that what is necessary on the part of all concerned with the problem of the alcoholic is to work together, and when we find areas where there are differences needing correction that they be corrected.

Question for Marty Mann: Has harm been done in calling alcoholism a disease? Would we be more honest if we called it a symptom of many diseases? Does the label "alcoholic" prevent getting help?

Answer: Let me start with the last one, does the label "alcoholic" prevent people from getting help. Yes, I think it does. I think this has unfortunately become a label of opprobrium—that some people would do almost anything to avoid having it pinned on them. Also I find a great tendency in people speaking on this subject, particularly professional people, in talking about somebody becoming alcoholic or being alcoholic to use "alcoholic" as a noun, grammatically as the subject of a sentence—meaning a person, a person who has a particular condition. If, however, "alcoholic" is reserved for its primary grammatical usage as an adjective, then the word they should be using is "alcoholism," which can function as the object of the sentence to describe what the person *has,* not to accuse him as to what he *is.*

The point is subtle, and can be illustrated by a suggestion made many years ago by a student and teacher in this field who happens to be a Jesuit. Maybe you'll think this is a typical Jesuitical suggestion. I don't know. But it is an interesting experience that this man had. He was Professor of Moral Theology at a Catholic University and therefore had considerable position, you might say, particularly among the Catholic families of the community. One of the families had an alcoholic member on whom a great deal of money and time and effort had been spent. It was the wife and mother in the family, and she had been hospitalized many times and sent to many institutions. She had been sent to many doctors and nothing apparently had done any good. At any rate she was still drinking. In desperation the family asked this Jesuit priest to come in and talk to her. They were very good Catholics and they thought he might have the power to persuade her. Naturally to him, as she had to everyone else, she denied that drinking was any problem. And as she went on denying it, he somewhat exasperatedly said to her, "Why is it so difficult for you to admit that you have alcoholism?" She said, "What did you say?" He repeated it. "I have alcoholism," she said, "Why didn't somebody say so!" He elaborated on what had happened: The finger of guilt pointing at her with "You are an alcoholic" had shifted just a little when he said, you *have* alcoholism. Alcoholism became something that had happened to her, for which she was not wholly responsible, and she could admit to it without entirely losing face. He made a suggestion at one of the refresher courses in the summer school of alcohol studies that we all try using this, that conceivably this was a therapeutic tool, that this might remove some of the psychological resistance of the alcoholic to admitting being an alcoholic.

We at the National Council have talked of this a good deal, and we thought the point had validity and that we would attempt in releases, literature and talk to speak of people having alcoholism or people with alcoholism rather than always saying alcoholics. Instead of saying that someone is becoming an alcoholic, we say they are developing alcoholism. People in the field of psychiatry should recognize the great importance of semantics in therapeutic relationships. This word alcoholic has been used in such a way that it has become a whip, a finger of blame, pointing. It has become a sign of opprobrium; it has become a word that no decent person wants to be associated with. The alcoholic who is not quite ready to throw his decency overboard and say, "I'm just a bum and no good," is not easily going to accept that term. In one of the sessions of this conference a therapist in the discussion pointed out that he very rarely insisted that a patient admit being an alcoholic at the beginning. He didn't care what they called it. If they merely said they had a problem with drinking that was all that was necessary. I believe we don't think enough about the effect of words. I have been one of those who have wished that some other word would be invented to describe this illness and its victims so that we could get away from the unfortunate associations surrounding the word alcoholic and the word alcoholism. But no such satisfactory word has been devised.

Comment by Dr. Ditman: The use of the concept that alcoholism is a disease often takes one label and forgets the rest of the individual. Whether you think of it as a disease or not, you can make this mistake, that is, forgetting that the individual is drinking for some reason. This reason may vary with individuals considerably. Some people may have psychiatric problems underlying the drinking that need treatment more than just the drinking. So by talking of alcoholism as a disease one may convey the idea to some that if they stop drinking you are curing their alcoholism. For example, occasionally I see women in their late 30's or early 40's who are having a problem with alcohol, drinking excessively. The "alcoholism" or the drinking can be stopped, the isolation that has developed, the estrangement from their husband or family, these may go untreated. They have stopped drinking, and they may think, and the family may think that now it's all well. But something happens, depression, suicide, or maybe a divorce takes place, which might have been avoided. So, just to take the one label of alcoholism may be a way of overlooking what's going on in an individual.

Dr. Bennett: With respect to this criticism of alcoholism as a disease concept, we have many conditions we call diseases, which do not show themselves in terms of pathological and structural or anatomical changes in the body. It seems to me it is all a question of what we mean by disease. These are the sickest people we possibly can treat. They are very ill, the questions of semantics as to an illness, disorder, syndrome or whatever you call it is unimportant. I don't see the point in quarreling so much about the concept of whether alcoholism is a disease. It is a very disabling malignant sickness. It is probably the third cause of death, right behind cancer and heart diseases, if we had the true facts.

Summation

Mrs. Marty Mann: I'd like to go back to the basic subject we were discussing, which is how to get better relationships between not just medicine, psychiatry and AA, but perhaps among all of the groups and individuals whom we need to involve in solving this problem, at least in making a beginning toward solving the problem. I don't think we are limited, frankly, to the three groups mentioned. We have medicine, we have psychiatry, we have AA, we have professional social work, we have psychologists, we have the clergy. As a matter of fact we have a good many people in industry who are showing recently that they have a part in this. They may be personnel people, or they may be in medical departments, although they may not themselves be doctors. I think, too, that we have society as a whole in which people live. Alcoholics don't live in a vacuum. They live among all of us. It seems to me that the broadest possible concept of the therapeutic community is what we must have if we are really going to solve the alcoholism problem. So I think we have to get better relationships all around. I think there must not only be an understanding, an increasing understanding, and cooperative relationships between psychiatry, medicine, AA and the yet untreated alcoholic population, but, because the largest majority of our alcoholics are still untreated, because less than 10% of them have been brought to any kind of treatment and have recovered, I think we have to extend this relationship, this cooperative relationship, this understanding of what everyone can do throughout the community. This is the work that the National Council on Alcoholism is trying to do. This is our objective when we help a community to organize a Council on Alcoholism, whose objective is to involve the total community in doing something about the problem of alcoholism. Now if you are going to involve them they've each got to understand where the other one sits. What is the involvement necessary on the part of these various groups that make up a community? What responsibility does each of them have? How much of that responsibility are they taking or could they take? All of this I think is important. Certainly it is crucial, right at the heart of the matter, to get better relationships between medicine, psychiatry and AA, because here are three groups that clearly have a great deal to offer and clearly can make a tremendous difference in the status of the present alcoholic population—if they are working properly, if they are working together, if they are all putting into it what they have to put into it. I also feel very strongly that this cannot be fragmented. It's not just that the person is a whole, but the community is also a whole, and all are involved. I don't think we can fragment this and say that this little piece belongs to you and that little piece belongs to you, now take it off at the corner and eat it and don't bother anybody. I think they all have to get together. This kind of thing, it seems to me, this type of discussion together, is the kind of thing there ought to be a lot more of. I think it has been tremendously helpful and I hope that its constructive and helpful aspects will reach out in all necessary directions.

Dr. Ditman: As Mark Twain says: "In all matters of opinion our adversaries are insane." In the field of alcoholism there are a great many viewpoints as to what it is. For example, at a recent meeting, investigators from different parts of the country sat down to decide what alcoholism was and produced nine different positions. In view of our lack of knowledge of alcoholism there is a great deal of room for differences of opinion. There are many approaches that can be used. I don't think we need to think that are adversaries are insane; I think we should learn to respect these differences of opinion and work together. I think ultimately as we get more facts about alcoholism we can do more with it and we will have fewer differences of opinion. I think that this is taking place now, and should be encouraged. Cooperation between professional groups, paramedical groups and lay groups is needed. Much more needs to be done in the training of specialists in treatment of alcoholism. It is, I think, a sad fact that our own Psychiatric Association at the present doesn't have a committee on alcoholism. I understand and hope that one is going to be formed. That is also true of our local Southern California Psychiatric Association. Let me end on an optimistic note: At least we had two meetings tonight on alcoholism.

Dr. Paul O'Hollaren: I, too, would like to end on an optimistic note. I think we have very definite signs of progress. I have worked very hard on this problem for 24 years and only succeeded in treating 12,000 cases in that time. During those same twenty years, in the statistics that Dr. Bennett quoted, there have been 4,000,000 new alcoholics develop. So I'm losing ground. It seems to be much more intelligent and much more effective for all of us to look for the prevention of this disease than try to keep picking up these broken bodies and try to put them back together. I think none of us is spending enough time looking at the basic cause, being realistic about what really causes this disease, and that is alcohol. I think more research around the effects of alcohol is very much overdue—and not in just the animal. I think there is a bad lack of communication. We have to get the medical group, the psychiatric group, the AA, and people involved in law enforcement and legislative forces together. If we just sit around without putting our heads together, how are we ever going to get any programs in front of the people who are in a position to do something about the problem. As a unified force we could get something done.

Dr. Voldeng: With the illness alcoholism, we are dealing with a very unusual and unique situation. I think it makes little difference whether you call it an illness, a behavior disturbance, a psychoneurosis, or whatever you want to tag it, the fact is that the sequence of events has a morbidity, mortality, cause, and treatment. We have been side-stepping, disregarding, and neglecting this seriously handicapped and doomed individual for many years. Not only the doctors, but the clergy, police officers, and all segments of society are equally guilty. It was AA that actually awakened us and brought about some understanding of the alcoholic individual. It was AA that proved to the world that the drunk was not hopeless in our society.

I am well aware that there is a bit of a gulf separating medicine and AA. How such a separation between the workable philosophy of AA and the scientific minds of medicine come about can be explained. Members of AA understand alcoholic behavior and compulsive drinking patterns. They quite understandably are amazed as they watch many of our profession misunderstand the alcoholic, fumble with incorrect attitudes and display our dearth of favorable results.

Recently the medical men have been seriously trying to learn more about the condition and to better understand the alcoholic patient. Even the psychiatrists who have done their share of fumbling are now doing a better job. The same can be said of the clergy.

I am convinced that all of us can help with this immense problem. I don't think that it is all the responsibility of any one group. We can all add our help, we can cooperate with each other, and I see no reason that a separation between AA, the Church, and the medical profession should occur. Most certainly, this matter of alcoholism is a serious medical-sociological problem. It is deserving of strenuous corrective efforts by our clergy, our religious institutions, our social workers, peace officers, medical men, hospitals, state institutions, in fact, every segment of society. I think we all are doing a better job. I think we are all trying to join in a combined effort. We have much to learn and a long way to go, but I believe we are on the right track.

Dr. Bennett: I would like to close with these suggestions. The principal reorientation in medical concepts of rehabilitation of the alcoholic will have to come, principally, from the family physician. Only the physician can give the friendly acceptant attitude that can reassure sick patients. He can best strengthen the motivation of the weak person to want to stay sober and the mental discipline to refuse the first drink. A physician has to become informed of a compulsive addictive disorder and be aware of the step by step process of rehabilitation. He can eliminate his frustration and impatience by understanding the alcoholic as a sick person. He must accept his hostile, antagonistic attitude as evidence of his illness, in the same way as we accept the disagreeable attitude of the psychopathic actor outer, the unreasonable neurotic, or the fixed unchangeable attitude of the paranoid or hypochondriac. The doctor must learn that many of these traits are due to organic brain damage and may clear with proper treatment. We have to treat all these people and accept their attitudes. We must likewise learn to overcome our prejudice and not reject the sick alcoholic. The family doctor should learn all he can about the great help obtainable through Alcoholics Anonymous, inform patients and encourage them to take full advantage of this resource, even personally calling AA to meet reluctant patients. We need to know when psychiatric referral is indicated, as, for example, in persistent anxiety states that need special individual psychotherapy. The challenge to better medical care of the alcoholic is a very real one and should interest every physician.* Thank you all for your interest and contributions. I am sure you all agree that Marty Mann richly deserves her honorary fellowship in the Psychiatric Association for her outstanding contributions.

* To get more younger physicians training in alcoholism, my Foundation has been giving annual scholarship grants through the American Medical Association on Alcoholism. These pay all expenses of the summer school at Rutgers University. Almost all graduates are active in research and rehabilitation programs.

CHAPTER EIGHT

Rehabilitation and Treatment of Acute and Chronic Alcoholism of the Brain

In approaching the subject of rehabilitation and treatment of alcoholic brain disease, I have chosen to start in a negative way by discussing first the reasons for failure in the treatment of alcoholism. This is because we have to better understand the complex problems that must be managed to effect so-called cures or rehabilitation. There is little sense or rationale for the simplistic approach to treating symptoms—a revolving door approach to alcoholism—and never getting at the basic problems or causes of the disease. Patching up an acute alcoholic in a withdrawal episode or delirium without proceeding to a complete evaluation and a comprehensive long-term program to obtain motivation toward complete sobriety is just not practicing good medicine. The disease is progressive, and, without intervention, relapse is almost certain to occur, with further physical and mental deterioration. There will never be enough dedicated doctors to treat the ten million problem drinkers and their steadily increasing numbers. The real challenges lie in more research into ways of early detection and treating alcoholism-prone individuals in a preventive program.

Failure to grasp this broad concept of the problem is illustrated by the criticism that I sent to the corresponding editor of the *Archives of General Psychiatry.* I consider this of sufficient importance to quote my complete letter. This letter was not answered.

> I would like to offer the following criticism of the article, "Revolving door alcoholic, an impasse in the treatment of the chronic alcoholic," by Drs. D. M. Gallant, M. P. Bishop, and co-authors; Archives of General Psychiatry, Vol. 28, pg. 633–635, May, 1973. This article was quoted at length in American Psychiatric Newsletter, giving the impression of an authoritative study. The analysis of 210 chronic skid row alcoholics and reasons for failure seems to me to have a serious fault. No mention is made of the chronic alcoholic having an addictive disorder, namely the compulsive, uncontrollable desire to drink, and the reasons for the inability to maintain abstinence. In other words, alcoholism as a disease entity. No mention is made of any investigative efforts to determine the degree of brain damage, yet they found 44% suffered serious physical problems. Treatment consisted of enforced group therapy for outpatients compared with compulsive inpatient group therapy along with adequate medical therapy (that was not defined) and attempts at social rehabilitation.
>
> The oversight in the project seems to me to be the failure to treat the disease of chronic alcoholism and the first requirement would be an evaluation of the degree of brain damage by clinical, neurological, electroencephalographic and psychological testing for organicity. In advanced brain damage cases, other neurologic evaluation to

determine the degree of cerebral atrophy, for example pneumoencephalography, would be indicated. Treatment with enforced abstinence from alcohol by the use of Disulfiram control until all evidence of brain damage is reversed. Then followed up by group therapy (including, wherever possible, Alcoholics Anonymous programs) and other indicated socio-economic rehabilitative procedures wherever complete motivation could be established, would in my opinion change the gloomy prognosis in a sizable group who would have reversible brain damage. There would be a residual group with irreversible brain damage and these should be permanently removed from society under some form of involuntary commitment to reduce the expense of the revolving door and protect the individual from his uncontrollable, compulsive progressive addictive drug disorder.

We and others have been extensively studying the effects of brain damage from alcohol over the past twenty-five years and have been able to salvage a large number of patients from their progressive fatal disease. References to a few of our studies are given below.

The authors call for early diagnosis and compulsory treatment but state there is no adequate prognostic clinical or psychological test data to identify skid row alcoholics and call for more research efforts toward adequate early diagnosis. I contend there is no such thing as a clinical entity of skid row alcoholic. The large majority are suffering from organic brain disease and if approached from this standpoint we do have adequate diagnostic and prognostic criteria but I agree much more research needs to be done. Too much emphasis has been placed upon looking at chronic alcoholism etiologically from the purely social psychogenic point of view and we need to get on with more research into the effects of alcoholism upon cerebral functioning and the resulting behavioral disorders.

Reasons for Failure

With the establishment of the National Institute on Alcoholism and a comprehensive alcohol abuse and prevention rehabilitation act, a great step forward has been made. The recent enactment of comprehensive alcohol abuse and the prevention-treatment-rehabilitation act is a landmark measure in meeting the problem. Also, leading insurance companies are giving some insurance coverage, providing the medical model of alcoholism treatment a great chance of succeeding. However, the National Council on Alcoholism (issue 39, June 6, 1974) submitted a report by James Kemper to the Ways and Means Committee of the U.S. House of Representatives, a national health insurance task force study. The purpose was to determine what forms of treatment were working, and to recommend specific insurance programs for adequate treatment. Among the problems uncovered were that:

1) Most medical doctors are unable to diagnose, understand or adequately treat alcoholism.

2) Hospitalization is expensive and not effective because no aftercare treatment essential to recovery is provided.

Better understanding of the principle reasons for failures in treating alcoholism would help physicians in the rehabilitation of alcoholics.

Since social drinking is culturally acceptable in western civilization, social drinkers have great difficulty in understanding the problem drinker, believing that alcoholic control is purely a matter of the will. They cannot understand dependent, compulsive, uncontrolled drinking, and they fail to realize that 10 per cent of drinkers are problem drinkers who become progressively addicted. This group, which is increasing in the United States at the rate of 200,000 yearly, is of major concern.

Much more effective public education is necessary if prevention and treatment of alcoholism are to succeed. People must learn where to go for information and how to persuade alcoholics to accept treatment. The 72 Alcoholism Information Centers in the larger cities (set up by the National Council on Alcoholism), as well as county and state clinics are available for help. Until there is widespread knowledge of the nature and extent of alcoholism, the alcoholic will continue to suffer social ostracism and disgrace.

Despite the American Medical Association's resolution that alcoholism is a disease, the medical profession largely ignores the problem. The fact that alcoholism probably ranks third as a cause of death should provide a sufficient challenge to them.

Psychiatrists generally have relied too much upon psychodynamic mechanisms in explaining alcoholism primarily as an emotional disorder, with psychotherapy as the main treatment. Too many believe that all alcoholics are of psychogenic emotional origin, ignoring the addictive, compulsive personality types who have become alcoholics just from excess use of alcohol. Many do not know that alcohol damages the emotional and intellectual centers of the brain, thus changing the personality. Constant excessive drinking produces a progressive cortical atrophy of the frontal lobes.

These organic changes, often subtle in nature, are treated as neurotic symptoms instead of as organic brain syndrome symptoms. Thus, patients still progress in their disease even while undergoing psychological therapy. Many alcoholics become disillusioned by psychiatric treatment and conclude that the physician does not understand the problem.

Psychiatrists need more training in their residency period to utilize all adjunctive techniques: medical and Alcoholics Anonymous (AA), along with psychotherapy. Nonpsychiatric practitioners must learn to recognize that an intolerant, nonsympathetic attitude can arouse feelings of anger, futility or disgust, which prevent the establishment of a working rapport. They can learn much from AA about how to establish a sympathetic yet therapeutic attitude.

Failure in Psychotherapy

Psychotherapy has been found to be ineffective for the following reasons:

Too many psychiatrists consider all alcoholics neurotic; the uncovering type of therapy is useless until the patient has achieved sobriety; many psychiatrists refuse to work with the spouse and/or others close to the patient; many alcoholics have no confidence in psychiatric therapy and are fearful of "insanity" or commitment; many psychiatrists have no personal experience with problem drinkers and are prejudiced, gullible and easily fooled by the alcoholic; patients often feel—and AA members confirm the idea—that a nonalcoholic can never understand the alcoholic.

Successful therapy must include genuine friendliness, with presentation of the facts of the illness, and insistence that the patient make any sacrifice required in treatment. The therapist must have tolerance to stay with the patient in spite of slips, so long as he is cooperative and trying, and he must always be willing to enlist the aid of AA or any others willing to give supportive help.

Other Reasons Physicians Fail

Most doctors receive little knowledge of the diagnosis and treatment of alcoholism in medical school. For instance, any physician who tries to encourage an alcoholic to cut his intake to controlled drinking does not understand the nature of the true addiction. Other medical practitioners render emergency treatment or handle the complications, and then consider their responsibility ended. Such treatment only patches up the hangovers and allows patients to return to their former, compulsive, addictive pattern.

It is the doctor's duty to encourage patients to accept a complete rehabilitative program. While giving emergency treatment they have a unique opportunity to influence patients. Here a physician can provide a friendly, acceptant attitude that offers help; he must accept a hostile attitude as evidence of illness, the same as a disagreeable attitude from a psychopathic acter-outer, unreasonable neurotic, or the unchangeable paranoid or hypochondriac. If he feels unable to treat alcoholism, it is his duty to know the community resources available and refer the patient to one who understands such total rehabilitative treatment.

Doctors often fail to understand the compulsive nature of drug addiction. They must grasp the principle of the repetitive urge to drink and appreciate the fact that abnormal, excessive drinking is not a willful, conscious act; only then can the doctor treat the compulsive, addictive personality disorder. Unless he sees alcoholism as this type of illness, he cannot cope with it intelligently.

It is important that he understand how AA works—how by means of the 12 steps of this organization, the patient is taught to sustain sobriety. Doctors may best gain such insight by attending AA meetings and learning how to identify themselves with the alcoholic. Such association will help them to better understand the alcoholic and develop the indispensable, sympathetic relationship.

AA refers to the process of obtaining motivation as "hitting bottom," meaning that the patient finally realizes he has a drinking problem and accepts the need for help. The problem from here on is one of keeping the motivation alive, either through AA or counseling of the physician, or through psychotherapy if indicated.

Physicians should not accept the idea that the alcoholic must reach the stage of severe deterioration before he can be helped. They should be able to find a way to bring him to successful therapy and not wait until irreversible damage is done, whether psychologic, social or physical.

One of the most difficult patients to motivate is the one with a high degree of anxiety, who uses alcohol to relieve his intolerable tension and to avert panics. This mechanism, which can establish the compulsive pattern of drinking within a short time, must be understood by the physician; He must be able to assure the patient that he can learn other effective ways to alleviate excess anxiety without alcohol or addictive drugs.

Symptomatic Alcoholism from Psychiatric Disorders

Any neurosis or psychosis may be complicated by alcoholism. Some of the most difficult problems are encountered in patients with hypomanic reactions, depressions, schizophrenia and organic brain disorders. Certain types of epilepsy are markedly aggravated by alcohol.

Unless the physician recognizes these psychiatric disorders as causative and treats them after the alcoholism is brought under control, no cure can be effective. The most difficult and disappointing group consists of patients with sociopathic disorders, in whom character defects are longstanding and motivation is difficult.

When an individual gives up alcoholic indulgence, his defenses are lowered and an acute psychotic episode may occur, particularly if a latent psychosis was present before. Although any extra stress with sudden release of accumulated anxiety may precipitate a breakdown, withholding treatment of an alcoholic because of this possible complication does not seem to be justified.

Suicide with alcohol involvement is 50 times higher than for the normal population. Some commit intentional suicide under the influence of alcohol—often combined with sedative drugs, especially barbiturates. Probably an even larger proportion die from psychotic or neurotic depression with symptomatic alcoholism. Careful psychiatric evaluation of all depressed alcoholic patients should be made, and where suicidal potential exists, patients should be treated for depression as well as for alcoholism and carefully followed up for at least a year.

Suicidal desires may be aggravated when alcohol is restricted. A very high incidence of suicides occurs during the remorseful state following a binge, a time when alcoholics often ingest excessive amounts of barbital. Some commit suicide by such methods as reckless automobile driving, which may be either an unconscious or consciously deliberate attempt to make the suicide appear accidental. Some resort to firearms, while a few commit homicide and then take their own lives. It is a physician's responsibility to recognize potential suicides and to recommend treatment in a psychiatric facility.

Another reason for failure in the treatment of alcoholism is that many physicians do not understand alcoholic brain disease. It is not difficult to recognize the poor prognosis in advanced stages, such as Korsakoff's psychosis, but diagnosis of early brain damage in alcoholics is frequently missed and the organic symptoms are often treated as neurotic manifestations. These patients, incapable of exercising good judgment, have lost control; they cannot resist temptation and compulsively drink until they reach a stage of unconsciousness. Brain damage may be recognized early if the physician is alert in detecting personality changes, intellectual impairment, and carefully analyzes psychologic tests or EEG changes. Prolonged restraint and medical treatment are indicated until the intellectual impairment and emotional instability are reversed. Only then can reconstructive therapy be started and motivation with full cooperation achieved. To achieve full control of the patient, family cooperation is necessary. With such methods, large numbers of these patients can be salvaged who would otherwise deteriorate, placed in state hospitals, or die of alcoholic complications.

Missed diagnoses account for many failures. Many women drinkers continue for years until some complication forces recognition of an uncontrolled drinking pattern. Many are hospitalized because of complaints referable to the gastrointestinal or nervous system without the true etiologic factor being uncovered. Women with menopause problems—or with children leaving, problems of health, widowhood, lack of new interests—may develop dependency upon alcohol. The associated use of sedatives, antidepressants and tranquilizers hastens the addictive process.

A history from a close relative, if alcoholism is suspected, may be revealing. In patients with anemia or malnutrition of unknown origin, alcohol should be considered as a possible cause, since severe complications may occur in these patients. A bromsulphalein retention over 5 mg.% may indicate alcoholism. There is increasing evidence that many instances of cardiopathy are the result of alcoholism.

The etiology of delirium and convulsions is never determined in many patients. These often occur when the patient is hospitalized and alcohol is suddenly withdrawn. Only by uncovering the true situation and confronting the patient and his family with the facts can the patient be treated meaningfully.

An infrequent cause of alcoholism is undetected epilepsy. Epileptics, like patients with post-traumatic brain disorders, have a lowered tolerance to alcohol. Those with psychomotor epilepsy have profound personality changes and may experience attacks of unprovoked anger, with blackouts, or even commit serious crimes. Their condition is aggravated by the use of alcohol. In any individual who shows unusual, explosive, violent, or paranoid reactions after drinking small amounts of alcohol, an EEG should be obtained. If an epileptic equivalent is found, both the epileptic state and alcoholism should be treated.

Failure in Understanding Rehabilitative Theory on the Part of Patient and Family

The patient may be poorly motivated because of his lack of desire to give up alcohol; he may wish only to bring drinking under control, may fear to face reality; may deny dependency, and may lack insight (often due to brain damage). The patient may not be able to control his anxiety without using alcohol or other drugs; or may have chronic, partial suicidal desires; and may be unable to resolve hostilities without alcohol, which fortifies his courage to act aggressively. He may have a continued regressive desire to remove inhibitions, release euphoria and indulge in sexual aggression or infantile fantasies.

Lack of confidence in the therapist and inability to accept the disease-concept of alcoholism may also be contributing factors to poor motivation.

Those who become addicted, who do not wish to give up alcohol, and continue to believe that they are not dependent, must be convinced they need help to control their compulsive drinking, that only with help can they learn to give up alcohol completely. They must become willing to make any sacrifice in order to achieve this goal, which includes cooperating fully with all prescribed therapy, whether AA fellowship, medicine, psychiatry or religion.

The therapist must be completely honest with the patient, yet not permit the patient to manipulate him. Even after the alcoholic expresses complete willingness to accept treatment, the therapist should continue all necessary controls and therapies to prevent relapse. Continuous, rigid controls are of the greatest importance until the motivation is sustained.

A prevalent misconception is that an alcoholic cannot be helped unless he seeks help, and is voluntarily cooperative. However, many who are forced into therapy can be motivated to accept treatment. The hostile attitude may become less intense as the effects of chronic intoxication are removed and the patient begins to think more clearly. During the remorseful state, or hangover, a patient more readily accepts the need for treatment. Often, through the understanding attitude of the physician and through educational reading, the patient becomes convinced he has a problem beyond his control and will accept therapy. Even if forced through legal controls, he may come to admit that he has to face his problem and accept help. Too many physicians use the absence of voluntary compliance as an excuse not to accept the alcoholic. When the patient's history indicates serious addiction, then forceful measures to get him into treatment must be recommended.

Other Problems in Total Rehabilitation

A frequent cause of failure in maintaining sobriety is poor social adjustment. Those with limited outlets (no hobbies, no close companions, or those who live alone) find it difficult to change this pattern. Many are obsessional workers without social interests, who find their only outlet through alcohol. Unless one can come to grips with this aspect of the problem, relapses are bound to occur. The author has been most successful with these patients when they participated in an AA program. Many older patients, or those forced into premature retirement, fall into this group.

Some patients need individual psychotherapy in order to understand the reasons for their feelings of social inadequacy, their introversion, or sexual shyness. Where definite psychogenic conflicts exist, with new insight such individuals can build self-confidence and develop new interests.

Many failures in treatment occur because of marital maladjustment. Since the attitude of the spouse is a vital factor in the success of the treatment, it is extremely important to enlist the aid of this person. If the marriage is still intact and a good love relationship exists, the prognosis is much better. More often, however, the marriage is threatened, divorce or separation may have begun, and the patient comes under duress, hoping to save the marriage. If both man and wife are excessive drinkers, treatment invariably fails unless both are brought into a non-drinking situation. By working together, their motivation is reenforced, and if they are willing to enter AA, they can get great help in sustaining sobriety. If the spouse is non-alcoholic, then Al-Anon should be recommended.

A severe source of frustration may be children who have lost respect for the alcoholic parent. Patience and time are needed to work out the problems; in some cases, the parent must learn to accept permanent hostility.

Pastoral counseling, if the pastor has a thorough understanding of alcoholism, can be of great aid in working with the spouse and children of the alcoholic. When the spouse is guided until the patient becomes firmly fixed in a therapeutic program, the marriage may often be saved.

Too often the wife, or relatives, foster progression of the disease by failing to get the patient into treatment. Unwittingly, such a relative assumes the position of therapist and, not understanding the nature of the disease, errs in directing the patient.

The patients who are most difficult to treat are those who lack responsibility. Some have too much money and do not work. With an abundance of leisure, alcoholic indulgence may become the main pleasure outlet. With the absence of responsibility comes idleness, boredom, a sense of uselessness, and eventually depression. Those who value their work and feel a strong desire to hold their jobs are more easily motivated to give up alcohol. Others who have already lost their jobs may become motivated toward complete rehabilitation if hope can be held out that they will be aided in finding work; but they must get medical certification that they are maintaining sobriety and cooperating with treatment.

Changes in Attitude Necessary to Prevent Relapse

There is usually a great need for the alcoholic to build a new image of himself and to recognize that a new, quite different personality is emerging. The alcoholic must learn to declare openly, without embarrassment, that he cannot drink. The new image must bring too, the strength to face realities. Some expect too much emotional satisfaction in their newly found sobriety and are not prepared to face painful realities, such as the need to rebuild friendships, social esteem, and faulty family attitudes. If the physician has not prepared the patient to meet such crises, he may give in to disappointment and adopt a self-destructive, hopeless attitude—"I don't care, what's the use"—and decide to drink again. But if the physician is able to recognize the depression, he may pave the way and avoid the relapse. Counseling is needed over a long period to rebuild self-confidence and to get patients able to live with tension and frustration.

Other patients after a few months develop an attitude of self-assurance and believe that they no longer need followup treatment, whether by a physician or AA contacts. When the patient begins to let down his guard and is not willing to continue in therapy, it is indicative that he needs treatment more than ever. He still wants to drink and believes he can take one and quit. These phases usually occur in patients with cyclothymic personalities, who need psychiatric understanding to cope with the periods of elation or depression. During elated moods they are no longer worried, for their problems all seem solved. In depression such symptoms emerge as insomnia, fatigability, lack of energy, or merely low spirits. With patients who continue to believe they can someday again drink socially, therapy must be directed toward fuller insight. They must continue to receive medical or AA assistance; they must come to believe in authority, to realize that they cannot drink, to accept the need for a long-term recovery program, or to rely on disulfiram.

Failures in AA

Although AA has proved more successful than the medical profession in the treatment of alcoholism, it reaches only a small percentage of alcoholics (Chapter 7). Many alcoholics at first refuse this help because of ignorance. Others become disappointed by an AA meeting and fail to get proper orientation. Others object to the religious aspect of the program. The physician must be patient and await the appropriate time to discuss and overcome these objections.

Among the obvious factors which prevent the alcoholic from accepting AA is that he resists the idea of needing the total treatment program, and offers excuses to justify his position. Sometimes when this is pointed out to him by a physician or an AA member he will see the logic and will offer to cooperate. Sometimes it takes an unusual threat to health, or a socially unpleasant personal experience, to make an alcoholic aware of the seriousness of the problem. When he realizes he has a "monkey on his back" (addiction), conversion or motivation begins.

AA is often not the entire answer to the problem. It has functioned in complete isolation so far as medicine is concerned, partially due to the lack of knowledge and interest of physicians. Too many rigid AA members condemn medical and psychiatric treatment and encourage patients to ignore doctors' prescriptions for drugs, including Antabuse, thus often causing a relapse into further compulsive drinking. Many in AA believe all tranquilizers and sedatives are addictive.

Many members reject an alcoholic who cannot accept their philosophy, while others fail to understand the relationship between emotional disorders and alcoholism. The tremendous role of resentment and defiance against something or somebody has to be considered in any therapeutic program. Alcoholics, like other patients with emotional disorders, are seeking peace of mind. Some interpret a failure to remain sober as a lack of faith in AA, whereas the lack of control may be the result of alcoholic brain damage that needs correction before self-control is possible.

Improved communication between the groups is badly needed, for the best results occur when AA works actively with doctors. When AA members visit patients in the hospital, a better understanding invariably results and more patients are salvaged. Physicians experienced in the treatment of the disease have a responsibility to educate AA on medical facts, and leaders in AA should offer assistance to physicians and invite them to attend meetings.

Just as AA believes that an alcoholic must admit his own weakness before he is willing to seek help, so it is true in the psychiatric approach. As long as the individual believes in the strength of his own ego, he is not ready for any type of conversion cure. In other words, he must surrender (become motivated) and, with strong feelings of conviction, accept the need of treatment, thus admitting that he is unable to control his drinking.

The refusal of the addict to cooperate is not a willful act, but is due to unconscious attitudes and chemical dependency, true drug addiction. This brain disorder causes the compulsive, addictive personality disorder, which prevents the patient from giving up drinking through sheer will-power. Only when he realizes that the painful phases of indulgence far outweigh the length of pleasurable ones does he have an honest desire to quit drinking. When he possesses a real desire to substitute something more satisfying for the transient pleasures of alcohol, then he is a favorable candidate for medical or psychiatric treatment, Alcoholics Anonymous, or a combined program.

This shows the necessity of having a comprehensive understanding of and readiness to use all facilities at our command to aid in recovery. These include community resources, family cooperation, along with all medical, psychiatric and social modalities. The goals are first to get motivation, complete cooperation. The objective is to get the patient to want to change, and to feel that he can make a new life without alcohol and find real satisfaction in total and permanent abstinence. In this endeavor the physician in charge must know the community resources to which he can turn for help, social agencies and workers, family counselors, the clergy, Alcoholics Anonymous and similar group therapies, and education of the family as to the objectives to be accomplished. There must be close contact with the physician by family members for any sign of relapse and especially to see that the patient carries out all the prescribed therapies, drugs in particular, especially if the patient is on continuous Antabuse.

The goal is to assist the alcoholic to gain freedom from his abnormal dependence and to achieve total, permanent abstinence. This goal must be constantly foremost in the physician's and the patient's mind. The physician should never tolerate the notion that the patient can ever become a social or controlled drinker; he must use every means to convince the patient of the necessity for absolute abstinence. To accomplish this favorable readjustment in the defective personality pattern, all these factors must be clearly set forth, and this is the real role of psychotherapy in the follow-up program. The physician must make frequent checks with those close to the patient, not relying on the patient's word until he is confident that the patient is thoroughly motivated and completely honest with the therapist. One has to educate the patient to expect the process of rehabilitation to take a long time, perhaps a lifetime; since it required years to establish addiction, it may take years to acquire freedom from dependency.

Treatment of Acute Alcoholism

The first step is medical evaluation. Treatment depends upon the stage of alcoholism. Acute alcoholism, hangover, withdrawal or complicated delirium and hallucinosis always mean that hospitalization for detoxification is necessary. This includes psychiatric nursing, intravenous administration of glucose, saline and vitamins, with emphasis on nutrition, overcoming dehydration and restoration of normal metabolic reactions. A few acutely disturbed patients may require immediate sobering up treatment. The following measures have been helpful: rapid intravenous injection of a subconvulsive dose of Metrazol; 3 to 4 cc or one gram of Antabuse is found to bring about drastic improvement in violent, combative, acutely intoxicated individuals. I avoid as much as possible tranquilizers, antidepressants, sedatives and even phenothiazines, as they are of little emergency help, and some, such as diazepam, chlordiazopoxide, and meprobamates, are replacement addictive drugs for the alcoholic.*

I find that physicians tend to turn too readily to sedation or tranquilizers to alleviate acute intoxication syndromes. The Journal of the American Medical Association published some treatment studies recently which show that drug therapy was prescribed in 70 per cent of visits to offices or hospitals, on house calls, or by telephone to alcoholics. The main drugs prescribed were psychotropics, vitamins and barbiturates. In hospitals, over 90 per cent of physicians treating alcoholics prescribed major tranquilizers and barbiturates in the majority of cases, while only 6 per cent prescribed Antabuse. I see little merit in the common practice of giving large doses of chlordiazepoxide (Librium), recently recommended for acute alcoholic brain syndromes. Many of

* Ford [33] found 23 per cent of 139 hospitalized patients were regularly taking other addictive drugs, and over 10 per cent were addicted. Multiple drug addictions must be considered in treating alcoholics. D. B. Douglas (JAMA 230: 375, 1974), in a letter on addictive drugs in alcoholics, stated: "Inter-group association of Alcoholics Anonymous in New York found 75 per cent of entering alcoholics misusing barbiturates, amphetamines and other 'soft' addictive drugs." He blames physicians and misleading information from major suppliers for trapping patients into these multiple addictions.

these drugs mix poorly with alcohol because of their depressive action and I have seen delirium tremens with small amounts of alcohol in patients taking large doses of meprobromates.

Before we knew of these tranquilizing drugs, we relied upon chloral hydrate or paraldehyde for sedation. In cases of extreme restlessness, tremulousness with insomnia on the verge of exhaustion or convulsions, one single large dose of paraldehyde (6 to 8 cc) may put a patient to sleep for about eight hours, and upon awakening he may be relieved of acute withdrawal symptoms—if proper care of nutrition is also given, vitamins and intravenous glucose for hypoglycemia are administered, and attention to any medical complications is provided. The most important treatment factor is getting the patient back to proper eating by forced feeding, a high caloric diet and even the use of small doses of insulin.

Treatment after Acute Episodes

If the patient is temporarily sober, one proceeds with the psychiatric diagnosis and treatment of the addiction, with special attention to determining the degree of brain damage. If the diagnosis is true addiction in a chronic compulsive alcoholic, efforts should be made to get the patient to accept disulfiram.

Disulfiram Treatment: After the preliminary medical and psychiatric evaluation, one carries out additional laboratory investigative procedures such as electrocardiography, electroencephalography, Bromsulphalein liver test, and others if indicated, e.g., kidney function tests, in addition to routine urine and blood studies. Patients with poor functional results in any of these organs may be rejected for treatment with Antabuse, or accepted cautiously as a calculated risk, with the dangers explained to the family. If the tests are within normal limits and the patient is willing, Antabuse is given, 1.5 gram the first day, 1 gram the second day, and 0.5 gram the third day. Then the test reaction is carried out on the fourth day. The test reaction demonstrates to the patient what will happen if he attempts to drink. The test dosage, usually equivalent to 15 cc. of alcohol in whiskey, wine or beer is given.

Antabuse Reaction: Within a few minutes after the ingestion of alcohol the following symptoms develop (if they fail to appear, a second drink is given within twenty minutes): flushing, throbbing headache, respiratory difficulty, hypotension, weakness, vertigo, and mental confusion. In a more severe reaction, dyspnea, vomiting, sweating, thirst, chest pain, palpitation, hyperventilation, tachycardia and syncope occur. Respiratory depression and cardiac collapse can occur, with a large dose of alcohol, within 30–60 minutes. Needless to say, the patient feels extremely uncomfortable, apprehensive, with fear of collapse. This reaction makes a profound impression and is not easily forgotten. If supportive measures are needed, in severe reactions, a guide is checking blood pressure: if it falls below 80 systolic, oxygen inhalation (95% oxygen-5% CO_2) is given. Intravenous injection of vitamin C, 1 gram, ephedrine sulfate and antihistamines are helpful. With milder reactions, effects wear off in thirty minutes, and adjunctive measures are not necessary. The patient often falls asleep and is normal within an hour. One does not need to give the patient a severe test reaction, and if he is really motivated to take the drug, one may forego the test, but I recommend it in all doubtful cases. If patients have systemic complications, such as severe liver disease, hypertension, or cardiac disease, it should be given cautiously. When the subject is a calculated risk, patient and family must be informed and potential hazards explained. The risk of continued drinking must be weighed against the nominal risk of complications from Antabuse reaction. The first sound color educational film on the use of Antabuse was made with co-workers by my Foundation. It is available from the Psychological Cinema register of Penn State College or Ayerst Laboratories, 685 Third Avenue, New York, 10017.

After recovery, the patient is discharged with a supply of the drug and directions to take the estimated dosage for maintenance, usually 0.25 to 0.5 gram daily. If given at bedtime, it acts as a mild sedative. He is supplied with a card to carry that explains the use of Antabuse and gives the symptoms of Antabuse reaction, with advice to call the hospital if he becomes ill. Follow-up visits for psychotherapy and for checking the drug dosage are arranged according to the individual case. We have observed a few patients who could not tolerate Antabuse. A few had psychotic reactions [35] from too large doses or from preexisting organic brain disease. A few others who inadvertently got alcohol in food, in wine vinegar, for instance—had reactions. A study of 131 alcoholics, 90 of whom received Antabuse, was reported [34]. (Forty-one with serious psychiatric or physical complications were not given the drug.) Fifty per cent remained abstinent, 15 per cent were partially successful, about 25 per cent returned to previous drinking patterns or quit taking Antabuse. Ten per cent did not report and it is not known how they fared. Many other workers have confirmed over 50 per cent rehabilitated.

Early in our experience with Antabuse we made a report in our first study over a six year period ending in 1950 [34]. 250 patients were treated with Antabuse before the drug was commercially available. We were overly cautious at that time, especially with patients showing brain damage or liver disease. We also had a few patients develop psychotic reactions from overdosage [35]. These were the result of cumulative action with delayed excretion of the drug. When we reduced the dosage, we had no further trouble.

To illustrate the sustained action of Antabuse, I took the drug, as prescribed to patients, for several weeks. Then I discontinued it; after one week I took one martini and felt very uncomfortable, with a mild reaction—showing that the effects can last one week after stopping the drug.

My experience with Antabuse leads me to believe it to be the greatest single contribution to controlling addictive alcoholism we have ever had. I disagree—in most cases, as noted in the provisos above—with those who contend that the test reaction is unnecessary. I believe that the personal supervision of the reaction is vital; it performs a useful psychological function in treating the patient, making him cognizant of the consequences if he drinks and helping to motivate him toward complete sobriety. Also, many patients feel greatly relieved to know that as long as they take the pill they don't have to be concerned about drinking, they feel safe and grateful for it. No amount of explanation of the drug's action will take the place of a demonstration of its physiologic effects combined with alcohol.

We rely heavily on the social aids, e.g., Alcoholics Anonymous, and in addition education of relatives and friends to understand the alcoholic's problems and to keep up informed of his progress. It is felt that group psychotherapy offers much in the way of handling larger numbers of patients through well regulated programs. Opportunities to consult with AA members are offered to the patient while in the hospital, and each week an experienced AA supervises an orientation meeting, explaining the program. Such recruiting of new members in the hospital setting has been highly successful.

The Role of Psychotherapy

All alcoholic patients need some form of psychotherapy, but the orthodox psychoanalytic approach is of questionable value. Patients tend to relapse whenever painful unconscious material comes out. There are not enough psychiatrists to work with the massive numbers involved, so that more superficial methods may suffice, such as the use of social workers in clinics, group psychotherapy, and reserving individual psychotherapy to alleviate the more pressing problems. However, it is well to emphasize again that the problem requires all resources available in the community, and that all chronic alcoholics need support over weeks, months and years.

Consideration should be given to the proper relationship of psychiatric therapy to Alcoholics Anonymous (Chapter Seven). All patients with emotional disorders are seeking peace of mind and this is true of most alcoholics. They also have tremendous resentment and defiance against something or somebody, which any preventative therapeutic program has to take into consideration.

The author's experience is that little can be done for an individual until he breaks down and admits his own weaknesses and need for help. As AA stresses, an alcoholic usually has to hit bottom before anyone can reach him. As long as the individual maintains preeminently the idea of his own ego strength, he is not ready for any type of conversion cure. He must first surrender and accept help, with strong feelings and conviction and admission that he is powerless over alcohol. This AA concept differs from the average layman's viewpoint of a willful refusal on the part of the addict; and yet we know that refusal to face it is due to unconscious attitudes. Unless he gives in to this principle, the alcoholic cannot give up his drinking. It takes whole-hearted acceptance of his disability instead of half-hearted compliance.

The author believes the chronic compulsive drinker's search for pleasure is the basic root of his trouble. It accounts for his difficulty in honestly wanting to give up drinking. The addict is often relatively infantile in his emotional reactions. His addiction satisfies some inner instinctual drive and he tries to cling to the pleasure achieved by repeated drinking. Because of brain disorder, he drinks too much and falls in a stupor. He makes endless attempts to reach a state of continuous pleasure that always slips away from him. He keeps up his compulsive type of drinking until he gets into serious social, psychologic or physical complications and has to seek medical and psychiatric attention. Only when he comes to realize that the painful phases of his indulgence far outweigh the length of the pleasurable ones does he honestly desire to quit drinking, with a more normal reaction to his emotional responses. When he really wants to substitute something else more satisfying to him than his repeated alcoholic pleasures, he becomes a favorable candidate for either medical, psychiatric or Alcoholics Anonymous therapy.

Prolonged supervision along these lines will enable the cooperative patient to gain insight and gradually enable him to utilize his new aids to a more satisfactory way of living without alcohol. As stressed before, physicians must change their attitudes toward the disease to one of understanding and a desire to help, if the treatment is to be effective.

When Antabuse is prescribed as part of the treatment, one should never allow the patient to decide when to discontinue the drug but must rely on the physician's judgment as to when discontinuance is safe. One should expect the use of Antabuse to continue in small doses over a long period of time, in some cases over a lifetime. The physiologic antagonism to alcohol controls the chronic compulsive type of drinker, whereas purely psychological management is inadequate. I repeat, this drug is the most valuable adjunctive aid in the control of compulsive alcoholism available to us.

By following these principles in treatment, the addicted, early brain-damaged alcoholic will be able to find a new life without alcohol.

Treatment of Alcoholic Brain Disease

Psychotherapy is of little value while intellectual dysfunction from brain damage persists, as has been pointed out. All therapeutic efforts must be directed toward helping the patient rehabilitate himself. This means, first, complete abstinence to regain physiologic balance and reversibility of cerebral cortical effects. Even though our patients are informed of the seriousness of alcoholic brain disease, they are extremely difficult to treat, and many will continue, eventually dying of intercurrent diseases, or by suicide, or else becoming permanently institutionalized cases. If control can be established until organic symptoms clear and fairly normal judgment returns, insight can gradually be established and motivation to live without alcohol occurs.

After insight is gained, supportive psychotherapeutic efforts may be fruitful, along with other supportive measures, such as AA, to bring about sustained sobriety and effective rehabilitation as previously described.

The first consideration is medical care, often required for weeks or months, until the organic features of systemic disorders clear (anemia, malnutrition, liver, pancreas, polyneuropathy or brain disease). Education of the patient and relatives is important, and the significance of brain damage must be explained. Relatives become more tolerant of the patient's personality changes and unusual behavior if they understand that, through prolonged treatment, the organic features will improve. These patients require prolonged hospital control or close supervision at home to prevent access to alcohol until self-restraint can be established. To effect complete and permanent abstinence, the institution of Antabuse control, as previously described, is the only physiologic preventative we have. Here we usually have to enlist the aid of spouse or relative to ensure that patients take the prescribed daily dose. Once the patient accepts the routine, as a diabetic accepts the necessity of insulin, victory is almost assured.

During the convalescent phase, with insight obtained in the nonpsychotic patient, selected reading material to convince him of the seriousness of his difficulty and the need for prolonged psychiatric and medical treatment is prescribed. This also helps the patient accept AA, and arrangements are made to take him to a meeting and the stage is set for prolonged association and continuing psychiatric follow-up.

Because of serious hypoxic effects upon blood sludging, the use of anticoagulants has been recommended. Patients with symptoms of alcoholic brain damage are said to respond more quickly with a four week course of dicumarol. I have had no personal experience, but the subject deserves a carefully controlled study, including psychological testing of patients on heparin or dicumarol, vs. those on routine treatment, to establish definitely whether or not reversibility of brain damage symptoms occurs more rapidly under these conditions.

Other aversion treatments still have enthusiastic adherents; they usually are via emetic drugs to produce a conditioned reflex aversion. In the past, before disulfiram became available, I used this method but never was enthusiastic about results, as relapses usually occurred. More recently, electroshock and death threatening neuro-muscular paralyzants, such as succinylcholine, have been used. Such drastic measures have not been shown to be superior to other methods, particularly Antabuse therapy.

Prevention

For the first time (1974) Congress has passed legislation launching a 350 million dollar, two-year program for the prevention and treatment of alcoholism. The National Institute on Alcohol Abuse and Alcoholism will administrate the funds. Only a national, public health effort can ever produce an effective prevention program; this is the beginning.

Other Treatments Recommended

I use thiamine 100 mg intramuscularly daily, with all patients in acute withdrawal. If patients show an abnormal EEG or myoclonus suggestive of a convulsive tendency, Sodium Dilantin 100 mg, four times daily throughout the withdrawal treatment, is used. Phenobarbital is preferred by many as an anti-convulsant, but should not be continued too long because of its addictive qualities.

A study* recently reported on drug regimens for alcoholic patients was divided into four groups: Antabuse, chlordiazepoxide, multiple vitamins and no medication. Each group was checked at weekly intervals. Nearly all patients who were followed showed a high degree of sobriety: 85 per cent for Antabuse to 72 per cent with no medication. Those on Antabuse and chlordiazepoxide showed marked reduction of anxiety, while those on no medication or only vitamins remained highly anxious. The latter groups also had a high rate of drop-outs in out-patient programs. The best results occurred where there was close supervision and involvement in treatment by the physician, when rates of recovery were high.

---

* Rosenberg, C. M.: Drug maintenance in the outpatient treatment of chronic alcoholism. Arch. Gen. Psychiat. 30: 373–377, 1974.

Aversion treatment by emetic drugs or electric shock along with alcohol ingestion is used successfully because of the strong suggestive, reflex action. Most important is the physician's dedication to the treatment program and his ability to persuade and motivate the patient to accept the treatment. This element of the physician's job is essential to the success of any treatment method, even hypnosis.

Antabuse treatment is simple, easy to carry out and scientific as a physiologic antidote, definitely affecting the craving for and thus helping to break dependency on alcohol.

Some therapists in Europe have been using an intramuscular delayed absorption implantable preparation of disulfiram, claiming it is effective for six to eight months [36]. This method could be one way of controlling the severe compulsive addictive drinker who cannot cooperate on a purely voluntary basis (e.g., the severely brain damaged). Further research evaluation of the method will surely be forthcoming. Malcom et al. [37] gave 62 patients disulfiram implants and found that the blood level of disulfiram was transient. They believe the deterrent effect is psychological.

Lithium has been recommended by Kline [38], who has championed its successful specific effects in manic depressive psychosis. He finds that alcoholics on lithium had fewer alcoholic bouts over a one or two year period and seemed able to resume social drinking. He feels that lithium may be helpful in controlling certain aspects of compulsive drinking in selected cases. He thinks it changes the drinking pattern by directly affecting or countering the action of alcohol on brain cells rather than by diminishing underlying depression. I have had no personal experience with lithium in alcoholism but it is our most useful drug for treatment of manic depressives and allied psychoses and the associated incidence of alcoholism is very high in these cases. Sinclair [39] found alcohol intake decreased significantly after lithium was added to food in rats developed for high alcohol consumption. Further research is needed with large numbers of alcoholic patients and controls to determine the value of lithium treatment.

Fluids and Electrolyte Balance during Withdrawal Treatment

Beard and co-workers [40] studied thirty well nourished alcoholic patients. Total body water volumes, electrolytes, liver and hematopoietic function were studied in acute alcoholic withdrawal syndromes. Their positive findings were hepatic involvement in all patients, and chemical constituents were altered. They found increased water retention that reversed to normal in four days, and from this concluded that not all alcoholic withdrawal states are dehydrated and believe that routine intravenous fluids should be discontinued. They recommend the use of diuretics (furosemide—Lasix, 40–50 mg) as helpful in treating many patients. Patients with complications of vomiting, diarrhea or diaphoresis should be given intravenous fluids. They agree that 50 per cent glucose with vitamins is indicated in all cases, and that this produces diuresis. They speculate that isomatic hydration, the abnormal transcellular ratio of sodium, potassium and hypomagnemia, is involved in the pathogenesis of acute alcoholism. They do not mention blood sludging effects in the studies. This needs to be studied and considered in the treatment of fluid balance. Their studies are based more upon laboratory investigations than clinical work. I believe that each patient must be evaluated clinically and all systemic complications treated in getting the patient through the withdrawal phase. After that, his entire alcoholic problem must be evaluated and rehabilitation begun.

EPILOGUE

The massive epidemic of alcoholic drug abuse and increasing numbers of alcohol addicts is reaching intolerable proportions, seriously threatening our national character. The almost universal use of "the world's best tranquilizer with the worst side effects" should cause us to be greatly concerned. It reaches practically every family in some form.

My purpose in writing this monograph has been primarily to educate physicians to a better understanding of alcoholism, its serious consequences and how it can be successfully treated. I hope that it will also be of practical help to paramedical people who attempt to help the alcoholic addict. I have avoided discussions of moral, social, economic and other aspects of the problem and leave these to the sociologist and psychologist. My main objective here has been to get more physicians to face up to their medical responsibility in adequately treating the compulsive, addicted alcoholic. If the book succeeds in motivating more doctors to become involved, to take an objective view of alcoholism, to find satisfaction in rehabilitating seriously ill alcoholics, then it has been worthwhile.

BIBLIOGRAPHY

1. Bennett, A. E.: Diagnosis of intermediate stage of alcoholic brain disease. JAMA 172: 1143–1146, 1960.

2. Little, S. C., and McAvoy, M.: Electroencephalographic studies in alcoholism. Quart. J. Stud. Alcohol. 13: 9–15, 1952.

3. Lereboullet, J., Pulvinage, R., and Vidart, L.: Les limites de la desintoxication alcoolique. Bull. Soc. Med. Hosp. Paris 70: 527–528, 1954.

4. Courville, C. B.: Effects of Alcohol on the Nervous System of Man. Los Angeles, San Lucas Press, 1955.

5. Mayer, A.: Alcohol as a psychiatric problem. *In*: Emerson, H.: Alcohol and Man. New York, Macmillan, 1932, Chapter 2, 173–309.

6. Bennett, A. E., Doi, L. F., and Mowrey, G. L.: The value of electroencephalography in alcoholism. J. Nerv. Ment. Dis. 124: 27–32, 1956.

7. Lemere, F.: The nature and significance of brain damage from alcoholism. Am. J. Psychiatry 113: 361–362, 1956.

8. Lemere, F., and Smith, J. W.: Alcohol induced sexual impotence. Am. J. Psychiatry 130: 2, 1973.

9. Mardones, R. J.: On the relationship between deficiency of B vitamins and alcohol intake in rats. Quart. J. Stud. Alcohol. 12: 563–575, 1951; Williams, R. J.: Biochemical individuality and cellular nutrition prime factors in alcoholism. Quart. J. Stud. Alcohol. 20: 452–463, 1959.

10. Williams, R. J.: The gentotrophic concept in nutritional deficiencies and alcoholism. Ann. NY Acad. Sci. 57: 794–811, 1954.

11. Moskow, Herbert A., Pennington, R. C., and Knisely, M. H.: Alcohol, sludge and hypoxic areas of the nervous system, liver and heart. Microvasc. Res. 1, 174–185, 1968.

12. Knisely, M. H., Renean, D. D., and Bruley, D. F.: The development and use of equations for predicting limits on rate of oxygen supply to cells of living tissues. Angiology 11: 1–55, 1969.

13. Blomstrand, R. (quoted from Medical News): Liquor hurts liver regardless of diet. JAMA 4: 449, 1974.

14. Rubin, E., and Lieber, E. S.: Fatty liver, alcoholic hepatitis and cirrhosis. N. Engl. J. Med. 290: 128–135, 1974.

15. Naitoh, Paul: The value of electroencephalography in alcoholism. Ann. NY Acad. Sci. 215: 303, 1973.

16. Bennett, A. E., Cash, P. J., and Hoekstra, C. A.: Artificial fever therapy in general paresis with electroencephalographic studies. Psychiat. Quart. 17: 750–771, 1941.

17. Lafon, R., et al.: Findings of pneumoencephalography in chronic alcoholism. Rev. Neurol. 94: 611–616, 1956.

18. Tarter, R. E.: Psychological deficit in chronic alcoholics: a review. Int. J. Addict. 10: 327–368, 1975.

19. Dahlstrom, W. G., Welsh, G. S., and Dahlstrom, L. E.: MMPI Handbook, vol. I. Minneapolis, University of Minnesota Press, 1972.

20. Wechsler, D.: Wechsler Adult Intelligence Scale. New York, Psychological Corp., 1955.

21. Page, R. D., and Linden, J. D.: Reversible organic brain syndrome: psychometric evaluation. Quart. J. Stud. Alcohol. 25: 98–107, 1974.

22. Hathaway, S. R., and McKinley, J. C.: Minnesota Multiphasic Personality Inventory. New York, Psychological Corp. 1943.

23. Ryan, C.: Global amnesia: a dissolution of metamemory? (Unpublished doctoral dissertation) Berkeley, University of California, 1976.

24. Denerll, R. D., den Broeder, J., and Sokolov, S.: WISC and WAIS in children and adults with epilepsy. J. Clin. Psychol. 20: 236–240, 1964.

25. Wechsler, D., and Stone, C. P.: Wechsler Memory Scale. New York, Psychological Corp., 1945.

26. Rorschach, H.: Psychodiagnostik. New York, Grune & Stratton, 1948.

27. Costa, L. D., Vaughan, H. G., Jr., Levita, E., and Farber, N.: Purdue Pegboard as a predictor of the presence and laterality of cerebral lesions. J. Consult. Psychol. 27: 133–137, 1963.

28. Reitan, R. M.: The Effects of Brain Lesions on the Adaptive Abilities of Human Beings. Indianapolis, Indiana University Medical Center, 1959.

29. Thompson, George N.: Alcoholism. Springfield, Ill., Charles C Thomas, 1956, p. 457; *In*: American Handbook of Psychiatry. New York, Basic Books, chap. 58.

30. Marinacci, Alberto: Electroencephalography in alcoholism. *In*: Thompson, G. N.: Alcoholism. Springfield, Ill., Charles C Thomas, 1956, p. 484.

31. Bennett, A. E.: The effects of alcoholism on brain function and its relation to industry. Excerpta Medica, International Congress of Psychiatry, 1971, series #274, pp. 543–551.

32. Backeland, F., Lundwall, L., Shanahan, L., and Kissin, B.: Clinical correlates of reported sleep disturbances in alcoholics. Quart. J. Stud. Alcohol. 35: 1230–1241, 1974.

33. Ford, F. R.: Treatment of alcoholism, problems from substitution of other drugs. Calif. Med. 84: 20–23, 1956.

34. Bennett, A. E., McKeever, L. G., and Turk, R. E.: Experiences with Antabuse treatment of alcoholism in a general hospital. J. Nerv. Ment. Dis. 112: 393–400, 1950.

35. Bennett, A. E., McKeever, L. G., and Turk, R. E.: Psychotic reaction from disulfiram (Antabuse) therapy. JAMA 145: 483–484, 1951.

36. Whyte, C. R., and O'Brien, P. M. J.: Disulfiram implant. Br. J. Psychiatry 124: 42–44, 1974.

37. Malcolm, M. J., Madden, J. S., and William, A. E.: Disulfiram implantation critically evaluated. Br. J. Psychiatry 125: 485–489, 1974.

38. Kline, Nathan S.: Lithium antidote to alcoholism. Med. World News, page 45, December 14, 1973.

39. Sinclair, J. D.: Lithium induced suppression of alcohol in rats. Med. Biol. 52: 133–136, 1974.

40. Beard, J. D., and Knott, D. H.: Fluid and electrolyte balance during acute withdrawal in chronic alcoholic patients. JAMA 204: 135–139, 1968.